THE **IRISH DAD'S** SURVIVAL GUIDE TO **PREGNANCY** [& BEYOND]

About the Author

A regular contributor on the topic of pregnancy and fatherhood, **David Caren**, a Dublin native, lives in the Rebel County with his wife and three children. When he is not running his own company you will find him out running, often with the kids in tow.

More praise for

The Irish Dad's Survival Guide to Pregnancy (& Beyond ...)

'Just the book to see "Daddy" through.'
Maternity & Infant magazine

'We frequently get asked by our mums (and dads-to-be) where they can find information that's aimed at men about pregnancy and parenthood, and we're delighted to say we have found just the book ... A really wonderful resource.' mummypages.ie

'David Caren may become the male equivalent of Gina Ford, with every father-to-be hanging on his every word.' schooldays.ie

'A down-to-earth, practical guide.' Books Ireland

'Refreshing ... accessible ... Answers all those questions many fathers-to-be would never utter in the light of a pre-natal class.'
Sunday World

'A fantastic read!' *Mums & Tots* magazine

THE **IRISH DAD'S SURVIVAL GUIDE** TO **PREGNANCY (& BEYOND)**

DAVID CAREN

THE O'BRIEN PRESS
DUBLIN

This updated and revised edition first published 2018 by The O'Brien Press Ltd,
12 Terenure Road East, Rathgar, Dublin 6, D06 HD27, Ireland.
Tel: +353 1 4923333; Fax: +353 1 4922777
E-mail: books@obrien.ie
Website: www.obrien.ie
First published 2012.
The O'Brien Press is a member of Publishing Ireland.

ISBN: 978-1-78849-028-3

10 9 8 7 6 5 4 3 2 1
23 22 21 20 19 18

Editing: The O'Brien Press Ltd
Typesetting, layout, design and illustration sourcing: www.sinedesign.net
Cover image courtesy of Shutterstock.

The material contained in this book is not a substitute for examination, diagnosis
or treatment by a qualified healthcare professional. Facts and figures were correct
at time of going to press.

Printed and bound by Scandbook AB, Sweden.
The paper in this book is produced using pulp from managed forests.

Published in:
DUBLIN
UNESCO
City of Literature

Acknowledgements

Sincere gratitude to the fraternity of fathers who at first bolted at the idea of contributing frank and honest accounts, but who eventually succumbed – providing their surnames were omitted!

To Michael O'Brien, Susan Houlden, Nicola Reddy and my O'Brien Press family for their enthusiasm and continued support. 'What's up, Doc?' – Dr Tony Foley, for casting his experienced medical eye over my shoulder throughout the entire writing of this book and Lorraine Andrews, Lecturer in Midwifery in the School of Nursing and Midwifery in Trinity College Dublin for her invaluable contribution.

My thanks and appreciation also to Brian Byrne, Steve Boyd, Colin Cooper, Tracy Donegan, Tom Finn, Conor 'Ironman' Fitzgerald, Friends of Breastfeeding, Dr Yvonne K Fulbright, Jamie Harding, David Hickey, Home Birth Association of Ireland, Flor McCarthy, Miscarriage Association of Ireland, Brian O'Leary, Colin MacNamee, Lorcan O'Toole, PND Ireland, Ivan Santry, Ed Scow, Martin Thompson, Mary Tighe, Treoir, Paula Tunney and Dr John Waterstone of The Cork Fertility Clinic.

A special mention to a few of my dad pals who were always generous when it came to giving their opinion and feedback on pregnancy and fatherhood: Adrian, Bernard, Brendan, Darren,

Ian, Jason, John, Martin and Nick, and to the countless mums who were frank (too much so at times!) about what it was like having an expectant dad around during the pregnancy.

To my bookstore friends – thank you so much for racking it out, now if there's any space on the shelf be sure to face the cover out front! To Ted & Mags, aka Mam & Dad, for teaching me the number 1 rule of parenting.

To my gorgeous and supportive wife Ellen and my three wonderful and distracting children, who gave me a little time off from being dad to write about becoming a dad!

For E, R, A & D

Contents

Congratulations ...

Becoming a dad is one of the most important, life-changing events to occur in a man's life, one that comes with its own catalogue of emotions exclusive to expectant dads, the very centre of which is man's search for reassurance. Reassurance that whatever he is feeling is perfectly normal, that whatever he is going through other dads have gone through the same. There will be times when you will feel sidelined, out of your depth, powerless and confused. Including the accounts and experiences of other Irish dads within this book shows that any doubts or feelings you may have are all par for the course.

In early 2009, I launched dad.ie – Ireland's first website for Irish dads and dads-to-be. Watching over my wife's expectant shoulder at her flitting from one mum website to another, I quickly realised that there was no Irish home on the web for expectant dads. The popularity of the site led me down the route of bringing out the first pregnancy title for Irish dads. Having spent several years as a bookseller, I noticed a gap on the shelf for a pregnancy title aimed at Irish expectant dads – written from a dad's perspective.

The Irish Dad's Survival Guide to Pregnancy (& Beyond ...) is an easy, practical read, written by a dad for dads, filled with real accounts from a 'Fraternity of Fathers', expert advice and an array of useful tips that fall under the banner of 'iDad'. Words, terms and phrases commonly associated with the pregnancy feature as 'Bumpedia' throughout the book.

The Irish Dad's Survival Guide to Pregnancy (& Beyond ...) is NOT a book with page after page of comprehensive medical text, diagrams of lady parts, or any type of flippant laddishness which undermines the greatness of the event.

I do not suggest you rush through this book from cover to cover. Pop it in your locker at work, leave it on your bedside table or in the glove compartment in the car, dip into it when you can, and, in reading, try to stay a few weeks ahead of where your partner is in the pregnancy; this way you will be prepared as to what is happening next and how best you can help her and yourself.

During the writing of this book, I fell in line with the mystery surrounding the sex of the baby and alternated between the sexes in the text. Regarding your own relationship with the mum-to-be, I felt it best to play it safe and go with 'your partner'; after all, its definition does set the tone of the pregnancy: 'one that is united with another in an activity of common interest which affects *both* the parties involved'.

This is a very exciting time for you. I thank you for choosing *The Irish Dad's Survival Guide to Pregnancy (& Beyond ...)* and am privileged to accompany you on your wonderful journey. All that is left for me to write before you start on your new chapter is: Congratulations, you are going to be a *dad* ...

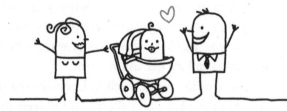

'It is much easier to become a
father than to be one ...'

Kent Nerburn

Introduction
You're going to be a dad ...

It All Started with the 'Late Late' Show
Tell-tale signs that she's pregnant!

'I'm late.'

   'No, you're standing right in front of me, dear.'

   'No, **I'M LATE, LATE!**'

   No other word repeated twice has the power to command man's full undivided attention, and no other statement has earned itself a more fitting response than 'how late?'

Something's amiss

More often than not, a missed period is a positive indicator that your partner is pregnant, especially if her menstrual cycle is as regular as clockwork. However, if your partner is not so 'regular', then she may notice other symptoms of pregnancy before it becomes clear that she has missed her period. While we are on the subject it is quite common that a light bleed (spotting) around the time she is due her period can be misinterpreted as being the start of her period when in fact it can indicate that she is pregnant.

Handle with care

If you catch her wincing when your hands gently head north, take note: tender, swollen and enlarged breasts are another giveaway that she may be with child. Tender breasts are caused by the surge of hormones in her body; the good news (for you too!) is that this feeling of tenderness does pass as her body becomes accustomed to the new hormone levels.

Make up your mind

Frequent visits to the loo are another tell-tale sign that something is not right, unless of course she has a kidney infection! Pregnancy hormones are the Jekyll & Hyde of babyland. One minute they'll have herself dashing off to the toilet more times than she can say Andrex, the next minute they're rendering your nearest and dearest incapacitated, unable to go at all. Unfortunately, constipation is not only a sign of pregnancy but a symptom which usually only gets worse as the pregnancy progresses.

Down and out

Lack of energy, tiredness and dizziness are other common signs of pregnancy. Feeling tired can be attributed to the change in hormones in her body, which usually disappears as her body adjusts to the new hormone levels. 'Hormones' can be blamed for a lot of the misdemeanours that occur in the pregnancy.

Is it something you ate?

Morning sickness is not a pretty or pleasant experience for your partner, or for the supportive gent who has to clean up the shortfall that didn't make the bowl, and though it can last the entire pregnancy (yikes) it is often one of the more obvious signs that your partner may be pregnant. While we are on the subject of what comes out of her mouth, what she puts in her mouth can also be a sign to start thinking about baby names. Keep an eye out for any unusual cravings – gherkin and chocolate sandwiches are a dead giveaway – and if she all of a sudden becomes repulsed by any of your favourite aftershaves and goes around sniffing the air like Teen Wolf, then it's time to pay the chemist a visit.

Stay positive

The home pregnancy test is the 'mother' of all pregnancy indicators. I'm sure, by now, you know how they work; it's not as if you put them in your ear. However, wouldn't it be nice to know a little more about the four-inch plastic device that can decide a man's fate in less than 300 seconds?

In a nutshell:
the home pregnancy test

Q. What do they look like?
A. A toothbrush without the bristles.

Q. What do you do with them?
A. ' You' don't do anything with them; your partner places the stick in her urine stream.

Q. How do they work?
A. They detect if a hormone called human chorionic gonadotropin (hCG) is present.

Q. When are they used?
A. At the time her period is normally due; however, more accurate about a week afterwards.

Q. What is the best time of day to use one?
A. Her first pee in the morning.

Q. How long do we have to wait?
A. Usually around five minutes, depending on the brand.

Q. What do I do?

A. Stay calm, yeah right! In the interest of fair play you could agree that, after your partner does the business to see if we are 'in business', she could replace the cap over the pee-y end and join you outside of the bathroom for the 'wait' – this way you'll be together when you go back inside to see the result.

Q. How do we know?

A. A result will appear in a small window with the word 'pregnant' or a symbol such as a plus sign, line or smiley face. Even a faint line is an indicator of a positive test. Recognising that this can be a 'testing' time for couples manufacturers have produced a range of digital tests that go as far as to spell out 'pregnant' or 'not pregnant'.

Q. How accurate is 'accurate'?

A. If instructions are followed to the letter and the test is taken at the correct time, then we are talking 1 to 2 per cent shy of 100.

Q. Can my partner be pregnant but still get a negative test?

A. She may well be, especially if she takes the test too early on in the pregnancy.

BUMPEDIA: **HUMAN CHORIONIC GONADOTROPIN (hCG)**

Pregnancy tests are designed to detect if a hormone called human chorionic gonadotropin (hCG) is contained in a sample of urine or blood. Also known as the pregnancy hormone, hCG is produced shortly after your partner's fertilised egg implants, or attaches itself to the inside of the womb (uterus). After this occurs, the levels of hCG rise rapidly, doubling every two to three days.

It is identified in the blood and urine within ten days of

fertilisation and, for this reason, forms the basis of all pregnancy tests. It is often suggested that a first morning urine sample provides a more concentrated presence of hCG, and that taking liquids before collecting a sample may dilute the presence of hCG.

iDad: **PEE LIKE AN EGYPTIAN**

Whilst many of my school pals opted to do mechanical drawing or art, I lined up for Classical Studies – it was a short line! Who would think that what I learned one day would come in useful for a book on pregnancy for Irish dads. Herewith follows a nugget of information that I learned during one double period of CS:

One of the earliest records of home pregnancy testing can be found from ancient Egyptian times. A historical document described a test in which a woman who might be pregnant could urinate on wheat and barley seeds over the course of several days: If the barley grew, it meant that she would bear a boy, and if the wheat grew, a girl. If both did not grow, then she would bear no child.

For keepsake!

You may as well know this now: throughout the pregnancy your partner may collect and save keepsakes by which to remember the whole experience.

According to a survey commissioned by the makers of the Early Pregnancy Test brand, the top three pregnancy keepsakes are ultrasound photos, items from the actual delivery (including wristbands and blanket) and finally the home pregnancy test which confirmed the pregnancy. Yes, you are correct, a USED pregnancy test. One can only imagine that it is stored away for when little Johnny gets married and Dad would stand up to say a few heartfelt words, pull out a suspicious pencil-like relic from the noughties and say, 'when Johnny was very small ...'

iDad: **IT'S A DATE!**

The actual day you both find out that you are expecting is an important date in itself, and one that should be recorded for future times, so to celebrate the date of finding out the news. Why not consider going out for a meal or buying a small gift for mum-to-be?

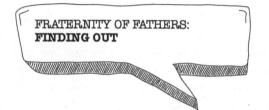

FRATERNITY OF FATHERS:
FINDING OUT

When my wife told me the news that we were going to be parents, I can honestly say I was hit by a wave of emotions the likes of which I had never experienced before. The range and variety of the feelings and thoughts that bombarded me was matched only by the intensity of the feelings. I have a number of friends who admit to the same experience. I have other friends who claim to have reacted with nonchalance when they were told. I'm not sure I really believe the latter group. The initial emotions were ones of absolute joy. As far as we were concerned, this was the greatest piece of news we had ever had. I remember thinking I would never have the same contentment as I had the day the news was broken to me. I was, of course, proven wrong when upon the delivery of my daughter I felt the same joy once again.

Darren, Dad of 2, Wicklow

We were on our holidays with all our friends and my girlfriend wasn't well on the journey over, which I put down to travel sickness, but on our first night over there she left the bar early to go back to the apartment. To be honest, I didn't think much of it until the next morning when I heard her throwing up in the bathroom. When she came out I was already sweating and not from the heat! We knew what we had to do, but as it was a Sunday, finding a pharmacy wasn't going to be easy. We eventually found one open at around lunchtime. Up to this point, we had to carry on as normal in front of our friends. When my girlfriend came out of the toilet with the test in her hand, nodding, my first reaction was to say, 'Did you just pee on that and now you're holding it?' Obviously this didn't go down too well and my girlfriend burst into tears. If I'm to be honest, I was secretly hoping that it was negative. We had both just started in new jobs and life was great. Now here we were on the second day of our holidays, with over ten to go, with friends who had no children of their own. We didn't tell our friends while we were there and, though it was difficult to take in at the time, we actually became much closer on our holidays. Two years on I have a baby son and I have to admit my life is better for it.

Tom, Dad of 1, Dublin

My wife came off the pill on our honeymoon. I thought it would be simple; in the next six months we would be expecting. It didn't happen. Our GP recommended we consider fertility treatment. After two rounds of IUI we became pregnant. I tell you, the day I found out was the second-best day of my life, the best being seeing the birth of my daughter nine months later.

Tony, Dad of 1, Cork

We had been trying for a while; my wife was meticulous in pinpointing when she was ovulating. She'd even call me in work to say to come home immediately afterwards. It all seemed a bit clinical to me, but I loved her so much and I knew how important it was for her to have a baby. The next time she called me in work, frantic, I cut her off, saying that I couldn't come straight home, that I had to work late, but this was not why she was ringing – she had just done a test and it came up positive. My first thought was 'damn, I wish I was there when she'd done it'. I seemed to be more overjoyed for her as it felt as though this was something she had done on her own. It didn't really hit me until I saw our unborn baby on the ultrasound scan; that's when I felt that I had let her down. I made it up to her throughout the pregnancy and hopefully afterwards.

Paul, Dad of 1, Roscommon

I remember saying to my girlfriend when she told me she was pregnant that I was too young to be having a baby. We had not been together long and I didn't know if our relationship would even go the distance. It didn't mean that I would just up sticks and leave her all alone either. It's been tough, but even though we are no longer together I still make sure my son doesn't go without and I see him nearly every day.

Michael, Dad of 1, Dublin

When my wife told me we were having a baby we were sitting in a restaurant in town and she'd just come back from the 'ladies'. She was very flush when she sat down so I put it down to the drink until I noticed she hadn't taken a sip throughout the entire evening. When she blurted out the news I can recall getting an onset of butterflies, then feeling very cold and then hot, then scared and elated, and finally emotional and dumbstruck – I didn't know what was happening to me. This must have all happened in slow motion because my wife left her chair to kneel beside me to ask if I was alright. I must have looked like a right fool. I will never forget the time and the place when I found out; my wife says she'll never forget the look on my face when she told me!

John, Dad of 1, Galway

IUI had worked for us on two occasions. We were very grateful and counted ourselves fortunate to have two great kids and so we decided that our family was complete. That is until one morning my wife – who was two weeks late, which wasn't at all strange really – announced, 'wouldn't it be funny if I was pregnant'. My wife had a stockpile of pregnancy tests left over from before. I can remember replying: 'only last week we said that's it'. Ten minutes later and our reflections in the bathroom mirror said it all – elated, astonished, disbelieving, confused but naturally delighted. When we told our parents they were not impressed at all that we kept it a secret that we were going again with another round of IUI. Safe to say, when they discovered we hadn't, they too were delighted.

Roy, Dad of 3, Dublin

Any father who has undergone IVF will testify as to how emotionally and physically draining it can be on your partner. A baby was the one thing most in life my wife craved; I would try to maintain a laid-back approach, in an attempt to apply a bit of reverse psychology, in the hope that my wife would not become too obsessed or frantic were we not successful on the second try. Inside however, I desperately wanted a child of our own, but I felt that I was better served reminding my partner that there were always other avenues we could explore if it didn't work out. When we discovered we were expecting twins I collapsed on the spot. My wife tells me I was banging the ground with my fists and crying at the same time. I have no doubt I was; whatever had built up inside of me needed to escape. After convincing my wife that this was actually a display of happiness, we booked a table in our favourite restaurant where we spent the whole night talking baby names.

John, Dad of 2, Kerry

BUMPEDIA: **THE EDD**

That very moment you find out that you are expecting can bring on a sudden mixed bag of emotions: excitement, apprehension, anxiety and uncertainty (as in, will we do another test?). When realisation eventually does settle in, one thing is for sure, you will both be desperate to know when it is exactly that you can expect to welcome your new baby (or babies!) into the family fold.

Determining the Expected Date of Delivery or EDD is often based on the last menstrual period (LMP) method. This method uses the date of her last menstrual period in order to find out when she is most likely to deliver, though bear in mind that our lady's menstrual cycles can be irregular.

The EDD is calculated by adding one year, subtracting three months, and adding seven days to the first day of a woman's last menstrual period (LMP). In other words, in the region of 280 days (40 weeks) from the LMP.

When you attend the first scan the obstetrician will be able to give you a better picture of the age of your baby, and therefore the expected date of delivery.

A Game of Three Parts

Trimesters

It doesn't take a PhD to figure out that the word 'trimester' has something to do with three parts. So when I tell you that in the context of the pregnancy that it means 'three months', I'm sure you are going to think 'well, that was pretty obvious'. Obvious it may be, yet it is important to note that each trimester will bring its own different emotional and physical surprises to your partner, and that as an expectant dad you will have your own role to play throughout the different stages of the pregnancy.

When we talk about a full-term pregnancy we are equipped with the knowledge that it is nine months, and therefore the concept of trimesters fits in quite well in describing that a pregnancy has a beginning, middle and end part – totally man-proof!

But since we are on the topic of matters relating to women, it's not as simple as it sounds. You see, typically a normal pregnancy is in or around 40 weeks long, which I admit is a bit longer than the suggested nine months.

In the case of trimesters, the first trimester is commonly defined as from conception to week 12, the second trimester from week 13 through to week 28, and the third trimester from week 28 to the birth. This can vary between 38 and 42 weeks.

Confusing it can be, and that is why I have steered clear of a detailed week-by-week analysis of the pregnancy and opted for the more expectant-dad-friendly three-part trimester guide, or more specifically: we've had the news, we're taking in the news, we have some good news ...

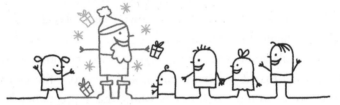

'There are three stages of a man's life: He believes in Santa Claus, he doesn't believe in Santa Claus, he is Santa Claus.'

Author Unknown

1 The First Trimester

Times they are a changin'

Trimester 1: Weeks 0–12

The first trimester is renowned for taking no prisoners. Just when you have stopped bouncing about with excitement with the prospect of becoming a dad, she starts crying and throws up on your good suit.

Womb with a view

A baby starts out as a few cells called an 'embryo' until it reaches its eighth week and becomes a 'foetus'– I know it sounds a bit too clinical so we'll stick with the name 'baby' from here on in. Your baby's development kicks off the moment the fertilised egg attaches itself to the wall of the uterus – this is called 'implantation'. Organs develop at lightning speed and will all be in place by the end of the first trimester.

Baby talk

'By the end of this trimester I can curl my toes, since they are separated, and I can shake a mean fist – both with their own set of nails, I might add. My kidneys, liver, brain and lungs are all working, but as I grow, they will continue to mature. You can make out my face, and my eyes have moved into their proper place out front. I can also close my new eyelids. What's that noise? Oh, that's my heart beating. I can snack on nutrients coming from my mum, but I'm not so sure if these 'buds' in my mouth that go on to become my baby teeth are of any use to me yet. Now, if I could only reach down, I could tell you if I'm a boy or a girl – you'll just have to wait for the scan!

'I have grown in size from a poppy seed to the size and shape of a cashew nut – we are talking cement block to skyscraper progression in the babyworld. Impressive, no? By the end of the first trimester I measure about 3–4in (7.6–10.2cm) long and weigh about 1oz (28g). My head makes up nearly half of my size. Just as well that I'm safe in a cushion of amniotic fluid, I wouldn't want to go banging it off something.'

Mum's the word

Expectant mums can sometimes be over-cautious when it comes to eliminating from their lifestyle what it is they feel may be a danger to their unborn baby. Her being pregnant does not necessarily mean that any exercising or sporting activity that she enjoyed doing prior to falling pregnant must be put on hiatus for the next nine months.

I have it from a very reliable source (Charlotte from *Sex and the City*!) that exercise is to be encouraged in pregnancy. Encouraging your partner may take the form of your own active participation in an activity such as walking, jogging, swimming, tennis, golf, dancing and cycling. If your partner is concerned about continuing on an activity, she would be best advised to speak with her GP or midwife.

Getting sufficient exercise and maintaining a healthy diet are essential in the pregnancy. Such a lifestyle will help to improve circulation, energy levels and sleep. It will also alleviate morning sickness, keep weight gain reasonable and reduce the possibility of postnatal depression. Your partner should also consider taking prenatal vitamins that contain folic acid.

The first trimester can be an exciting and daunting time for expectant parents: the first prenatal visit, choosing the right type of maternity care and the unfortunate worry of a miscarriage, which is more common in this period and leads many couples to hold off spreading their news until the 12-week safety marker.

Symptom sympathy

Due to the physical and emotional demands that being pregnant places on your partner's body, this will be a difficult stage for her as her body begins changing and adjusting to a growing baby. She may be feeling a tad emotional and tired. On top of this she may have to contend with heartburn, wind, indigestion, and possibly constipation. And just so she doesn't go thinking 'this is a piece of cake', let's throw in some morning sickness for good measure. It is important to reassure her that these symptoms are part and parcel of the pregnancy and 'most' will go away as the pregnancy progresses.

She may be hypersensitive to odours and flavours and may be put off by certain foods. Her breasts will be tender, meaning the area could be a temporary no-fly zone.

Shaping up to fatherhood

Pregnancy often presents an opportunity for men to get fit – like we needed a reason! We pull out the runners from under the bed and dust off the gym membership. Our baby's first view of their dad is not going to be as that fat lump cowering in the corner. It is safe to say that this new fit dad character may have a negative impact on expectant mum. Yes, yes I know what you are doing is admirable but be conscious of the fact that while one of you in the relationship narrows, the other – that being mum-to-be – expands, I mean blossoms. Be sensitive to her condition; the last thing an impregnated better half wants is a know-it-all fitness freak.

It may be time for you to make a few 'sacrifices' of your own and join in with the 'Musketeers' pregnancy programme. Intimacy may have to take a back seat for a while. And speaking of good health, research has highlighted that passive smoking can be just as dangerous to your unborn baby as first-hand smoke, which in itself increases the risk of low birthweight in babies, miscarriage, and Sudden Infant Death Syndrome (SIDS) or cot death. Show your support to your partner by limiting your own alcohol intake and joining her on her healthy-eating plan.

The 'All-Day' Infliction
Morning sickness

Consider a hangover without the consumption of alcohol, an upset stomach, a banging headache and the feeling of exhaustion for nearly three months. No, not some nasty strain of malaria, the better half has a case of **morning sickness**.

Although said to be an indicator of a healthy pregnancy (try telling her that when her head is down the toilet!), morning sickness is very common and will affect over 50 per cent of pregnant women, usually in the early stages of pregnancy, starting around week 5 with most sufferers noticing a reduction in their symptoms in week 16. Symptoms can vary from mild nausea to extreme vomiting, requiring hospitalisation in cases of severe dehydration.

Hollywood likes to portray the fairer sex as a type of superwoman throwing up in the middle of a crucial boardroom meeting, only to wipe her mouth with one hand whilst holding a 'coal and HP sandwich' (an actual recorded craving!) in the other, and still continuing on with business unaffected.

The reality is somewhat different. Morning sickness can stop your partner dead in her tracks, and assigning the condition a specific time of day gives it an even more cruel twist as it can strike at any time of day.

However, many of our partners will notice that it occurs at the same time of day and that they can, therefore, schedule their day's activities accordingly. There are various theories as to what causes morning sickness, including a change in the hormone levels, low blood-sugar levels, an enhanced sense of smell and sensitivity to odours, excess acid build-up and stress.

The following are various things that you can do for your partner to help alleviate the symptoms of morning sickness:

What you can do:

- Encourage your partner to take sufficient rest.

- Ensure that there is a dry biscuit or cracker to hand upon awakening. Your partner could try eating this before lifting her head from the pillow and then sit up slowly and take a small drink.

- Help with the daily chores, including the cleaning, caring for the children and especially the cooking.

- Make family and friends aware of your partner's symptoms and ask them to keep in regular contact.

- Avoid unnecessary conflict (throughout the pregnancy) and accept that intimacy may take a vacation for some time!

- Think of something different to do each week to take your partner's mind off her feeling of nausea.

When it comes to food:

- Buy foods that need little preparation, foods that don't have much odour, and be considerate and eat smelly foods away from the house.

- Provide small, regular meals or snacks throughout the day, to ensure her stomach is never empty.

- Avoid giving fatty, rich, or spicy foods and prepare bland meals, rich in both protein and carbohydrates and low in fat. A plentiful supply of carbohydrates will also keep her blood sugar levels up.

- Chewing gum and taking glucose sweets in between meals helps some women to reduce their morning sickness.

- Ginger is a popular remedy for nausea – root ginger especially, which can simply be grated into boiling water and drunk hot or cold. Ginger biscuits too as they tend not to upset the stomach.

- Top up that glass with fluids and ensure she drinks little amounts often. Ginger ale or herbal teas such as mint or ginger can be helpful (not too strong), but check with the GP first to see if herbal teas are acceptable in the pregnancy.

- Switch over to decaffeinated tea/coffee.

If you are ever in doubt of your partner's symptoms, consult your GP immediately.

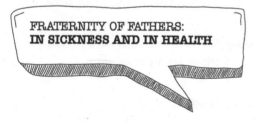

FRATERNITY OF FATHERS:
IN SICKNESS AND IN HEALTH

First of all, whoever coined the phrase 'morning sickness' should be slapped with a large wet fish. It strikes pretty much any time of day or night and varies in severity. Myself and the wife got off the bus on Bachelor's Walk and she starts feeling dodgy, most likely due to the fact that a certain old lady kept closing windows, despite my own and others' protests. No sooner were we off the bus than my wife darts a few feet down a deserted side alley and commences to get rid of that unwanted bowl of cornflakes. Now given that she is wearing a business suit and I'm casual but clearly not some junkie, you would assume that the majority of people would think 'PREGNANCY – the poor dear!' Not at all. It nearly came to blows with one particularly high and mighty 'gentleman' who felt it necessary to throw around comments like 'disgraceful' and 'Garda should be called'. I obviously defended my darling wife as she tearfully and emotionally threw up again.

Graham, Dad of 1, Dublin

Whilst holding hands, delighted to be out for the night and very much looking forward to a fillet, on entering the porch to the restaurant my wife turned white, signalling an onset of morning (evening) sickness. Thankfully not many diners witnessed the full-blown act, but safe to say the people queuing behind still turned away, even after being told my wife was pregnant. It didn't stop us having our fillets, though; well, I did help the manager clean up after all!

Jake, Dad of 1, Galway

There is a dustbin in the Blanchardstown shopping centre that will forever be a memorable stopping-off point for my darling wife when number two was on the way!

Adrian, Dad of 2, Meath

CATastrophe in Waiting
Toxoplasmosis

It sounds like a character from a Marvel comic book but toxoplasmosis is an infection which can be very dangerous to your unborn baby. Toxoplasmosis (or toxoplasma infection) is caused by a parasite, a microscopic organism, called *Toxoplasma gondii*.

It is quite possible that you, and more importantly your partner, has actually had a mild form of toxoplasmosis at some point in your life without even realising it; if this has occurred, your partner will be immune to the infection from then on and the baby will be protected.

However, if your partner becomes infected with toxoplasmosis, either while she is pregnant or during the 2–3 months before you conceive, there is a possibility that she could pass the infection on to your unborn baby, the effects of which may cause miscarriage, congenital defects, and damage to the eyes, brain or other problems. If infection occurs later on in the pregnancy the baby is usually born without symptoms; however, complications may occur later on. Symptoms are generally flu-like and fairly mild, but some infected adults have registered no symptoms at all.

There are several ways that your partner can contract toxoplasmosis, but cats are known to be the most common carriers of the parasite that causes infection. It is more typical in cats that are allowed outside and that may have fed on contaminated rodents. With this in mind, your partner should never change a cat litter tray as they are breeding grounds for the parasite that can cause toxoplasmosis.

It is worth noting that toxoplasmosis can also be contracted by eating raw or not fully cooked meat, and by eating fruit and vegetables that haven't been washed or peeled properly.

Don't be caught out taking a 'cat-nap' when it comes to toxoplasmosis:

- Encourage your partner to wash her hands frequently.

- Wash all cooking utensils and surfaces after preparing raw meat.

- Wash all fruit and vegetables, including ready-prepared salads, to remove all traces of soil.

- If you live on a farm, your partner should not handle lambing ewes, their afterbirth, newborn lambs, or the clothing of anyone else involved in lambing. Since toxoplasmosis can also be transmitted from sheep, pregnant women are advised to avoid contact with sheep during the lambing season.

- Feed your cat dried or canned cat food, rather than raw meat.

- Gloves should be worn in the garden. Take care not to put hands or gloves to the mouth, and wash hands and gloves when finished to remove all traces of soil.

BUMPEDIA: EATING FOR TWO

Pregnancy is the one occasion in your partner's life when her eating habits can directly affect another person. Your growing baby is dependent on your partner for getting a sufficient amount of healthy vitamins and nutrients to ensure that she has a good start in life. As far as the myth of 'eating for two' goes, it is not in the quantity of food that she eats, but in the quality. Incorporating fruit, vegetables, whole grains, and lean meat is essential to her diet and to the growth and health of the baby.

Take That out of Your Mouth ...
The no-no foods of pregnancy

A healthy, well-balanced diet is essential to the pregnancy; however, there are certain foods which your partner should avoid:

Iron woman: Liver contains a high level of Vitamin A which can be harmful to the baby. Similarly, pâté is also off the menu as it may contain the bacteria listeria.

Something's fishy: Shark, swordfish and marlin are to be avoided due to their high levels of mercury. Though tuna also contains mercury, consumption should be limited to no more than one fresh tuna steak per week or two medium-sized cans of tuna. Sushi and oysters are out.

Stay hard: Raw eggs may contain salmonella and for that reason alone should always be cooked fully. Take note of other food types made with raw eggs, including mayonnaise, homemade ice cream, custards and Hollandaise sauces.

Hot meat: Cured meats such as Parma ham and salami present a risk due to the possibility of listeriosis and toxoplasmosis. Make sure that all meat is thoroughly cooked and served steaming hot right through.

Oh nuts! If you or your partner suffers from an allergic condition such as asthma, hay fever or eczema, your baby may be at higher risk of developing a nut allergy.

Tipple time-out: Alcohol – need I say why not? Try to limit caffeine (tea and coffee) to two cups a day.

Dairy I say it: Drinking unpasteurised milk or eating other unpasteurised dairy products in general should be avoided, especially mould-ripened, soft, blue vein and unpasteurised cheeses. Hard, pasteurised cheese such as cheddar and Philadelphia are good candidates for the fridge.

BUMPEDIA: **FETAL ALCOHOL SYNDROME**

Alcohol can cross the placenta from the mother's blood into the baby's bloodstream causing low birthweight, infant flattened face, heart defects and developmental problems.

iDad: **FATHERS-TO-BE IN IRELAND NEED TO LOSE WEIGHT**

Two out of three fathers-to-be in Ireland need to lose weight; that's according to research conducted by Dr Ross Kelly and his colleagues at the UCD Centre for Human Reproduction in the Coombe Women & Infants University Hospital.

As part of the centre's research programme on obesity and pregnancy, under the supervision of Professor Michael Turner, Dr Kelly measured the Body Mass Index (BMI) in 167 men whose partners were booked into the Coombe for antenatal care. 'Of the men, 14 per cent were obese, compared with 16 per cent of mothers-to-be. In addition, 50 per cent were overweight, and only one in three had a normal BMI,' said Dr Kelly.

While the percentage of body fat was higher in women, as expected, the visceral, or tummy, fat was higher in men. Visceral fat levels have been positively associated with an increased risk of heart disease in adults. In addition, 32 per cent of the men smoked and 81 per cent consumed alcohol.

These findings raise important public-health concerns for men regarding obesity. Do men need pre-conceptual care? Is pregnancy a window of opportunity to advise men, as well as women, about lifestyle issues such as diet, exercise and smoking? Are public-health interventions more likely to succeed if they embrace both parents and the family unit, rather than individuals?

According to the researchers, minimising male obesity is

important not only for the individual, but also for his family. If he remains in good health, a father is better able to care for his family in the short-term and the long-term. If the father is obese, it is also two to four times more likely that his children will be obese. Breaking the cycle of obesity is important for future generations.

Won't He Feel IT?
Sex in pregnancy

Let's cut to the chase straight away: when your partner is pregnant, your sex life **WILL** change – I would like to say for the better, but in the majority of cases you should expect to have a less 'active' sex life during the nine months.

> **iDad: HOW MANY TIMES WILL YOU HAVE SEX WITH YOUR PREGNANT PARTNER?**
>
> Think of what your sex life was like BEFORE you found out that you were expecting, then minus the number of times you were having sex per week by three and there's your new figure – **for the month**! If you are in minus figures, then I suggest you get the clubs out!

I'm sure for most expectant males, you're reading this in bed, you have one hand on her belly and you're feeling good about yourself. The reality of the situation is just setting in as you move your hand away, only to be asked why you are in a huff.

But it's not all doom and gloom, and out of a famine some fortunate expectant dads experience a feast, with a small percentage of pregnant mums experiencing no change in sexual drive, and a few saying they actually have an increased interest in sex during pregnancy – you lucky B!

Expectant dads may also experience changes in their own libido throughout their partner's pregnancy. It is understandable to have anxieties and mixed emotions about becoming a father for the first time: the financial worries, the feeling that you may no longer be the number one in your partner's life, or that you may have sacrificed a degree of freedom that you had when it was just the two of you. You may also fear that sex may hurt the baby, or you may even be self-conscious about making love in the company of your unborn child.

Sex will **NOT** hurt the baby. In fact, in many cases, the motion of having sex will rock baby off to sleep. Rest assured your baby is safe within a cushioned amniotic-fluid-filled sac and unless you're having very rough sex, you have 'almost' no chance of injuring anyone but yourselves.

A lot of expectant dads feel closer to their partner during pregnancy than ever before (the fact that they can create a living thing makes 'man' feel all powerful and masculine!), and this closeness is often expressed in a physical way. For some, sex during pregnancy can be exciting (need I say bigger breasts), but for other men, well, it's literally a no-go area with some men finding the physical change a big turn-off. Please be sensitive – after all, this is the mother of your unborn child.

Your partner's sex drive too will yo-yo depending on what trimester she is in. She may spend a lot of the first trimester suffering from morning sickness, making her feel less attractive and desirable and less likely to engage in any type of sexual encounter, with the second trimester bringing in a renewed energy and heightened desire for sex. However, her sexual interest may dip again within the final trimester as childbirth nears and her body is at full capacity.

iDad: **IT DOESN'T HAVE TO BE 'BIG COTTONS'**

The top fashion houses across the world have started to turn their attention to the expectant mum market, offering an extensive range of maternity wear that is a far cry from yesteryear when women had to choose a few sizes up in their own clothes range to cater for expanding bellies and bigger boobs. Nowadays, maternity lingerie is making its mark

on the prenatal catwalk with many expectant fathers logging
onto specialist sites, buying up sexy (yet comfortable) little
numbers for their partners.

Getting into position

The way you have sex will also have to change. You may have to
try new positions (especially during the last few months of the
pregnancy) as your partner may find the missionary position rather
uncomfortable (bump) or too painful (tender breasts). Also lying on
her back is not recommended after the fourth month of pregnancy.

So which positions are most comfortable?

- It is best to try lying on your sides, either facing each
  other or by spooning (rear-entry position).

- The woman on top is also said to be the most
  comfortable of all as it puts no weight on your partner's
  abdomen and allows her to control the depth of
  penetration.

- Enter from a sitting position, with you seated and her
  straddling your lap, so she has her feet on the ground
  and can control depth of penetration and pressure on
  her body.

- On her hands and knees: a good position for pregnant
  women because of the lack of pressure on her abdomen,
  though some women find this difficult at the very end of
  pregnancy.

By all means experiment and find exactly what technique you and
your partner are most comfortable with. When you're trying to think
of a good position, try it, and if it doesn't work, stop.

Keep in physical touch with each other exploring other options
for non-sexual closeness, such as cuddling or massage. Or consider
exploring alternative ways in which the pair of you can feel close, eg
mutual masturbation and oral sex.

Oral sex is not dangerous during pregnancy (especially for men!); however, there is one exception – don't blow air into the vagina as this could cause an air embolism (blocked blood vessel) that could endanger your partner and the baby. Also, if your partner tastes 'different', don't panic – pregnancy hormones can alter the taste and scent of the vagina.

The use of sex toys in pregnancy is often seen as a taboo subject yet there is no scientific evidence that suggests whether their use is harmful or not during pregnancy. If using sex toys is a normal part of your sex life, there should be no reason why your partner should stop using them if she is having an uncomplicated pregnancy. The most important thing to note when using sex toys during pregnancy is to always keep them clean.

There are some important circumstances, however, when you and your partner may be advised not to have intercourse:

◻ A history of miscarriages.

◻ Unexplained bleeding, stomach cramps or discharge.

◻ Premature contractions that might indicate an early delivery (or indeed if your partner has a history of pre-term babies).

◻ Multiple pregnancies (with twins, triplets or more).

◻ Placenta praevia (where the placenta sits low and covers the opening to the uterus).

◻ You or your partner having an active sexually transmitted disease (in which case having sex will more than likely transfer this to the baby).

◻ Incompetent cervix (the cervix weakens and opens prematurely).

WHAT THE EXPERT SAYS:
GETTING IN THE MOOD

Some men have misconceptions about sex during pregnancy; others have trouble seeing their pregnant partner as a sexual being, or are suddenly seeing her as the mother of their child, which makes sex feel more taboo. Be supportive, even if you're not in the mood, as turning down sexual opportunities may have her more sensitive than normal.

Strive to maintain sexual intimacy that doesn't necessarily require all-out intercourse. Explore other ways to satisfy her beyond intercourse if you're not always in the mood. The goal should be to cultivate physical touch which acts as support for her and which nurtures the emotional bond.

Dr Yvonne K Fulbright is a sexologist, sex columnist for *Cosmopolitan* and co-author of *Your Orgasmic Pregnancy: Little Sex Secrets Every Hot Mama Should Know.*

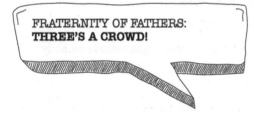

FRATERNITY OF FATHERS:
THREE'S A CROWD!

Your partner is the best resource when it comes to what is most comfortable. There will be a point during the latter part of the pregnancy where you might find that she becomes, shall we say, rather enthusiastic. It doesn't happen for everyone though.

Adam, Dad of 2, Sligo

On our first baby it was the one thing that I needed to know especially as I was worried about harming the baby. Not the kind of subject you bring up in the pub with your mates. But it turned out that the baby doesn't get harmed, so I would advise that you enjoy the new experience and use your ingenuity. But do so soon because from my experience, after another few weeks she might ban you from such activities altogether!

Jerry, Dad of 2, Kildare

It differs with each pregnancy so I would strongly advise when the opportunity presents itself, go for it, but be careful of the bump!

Patrick, Dad of 2, Dublin

What's up, Doc?
Well in advance of your new arrival

When the dust has settled and the news has sunk in, many expectant fathers turn their attention onto themselves. For the majority of expectant dads, 'responsibility' is a common word that crops up a great deal throughout the pregnancy (and beyond!). And not just in the manner that a father accepts that he has a responsibility to take care of his family.

The impending arrival of a new baby can tug at our health conscience. Getting ourselves into shape, watching our diets and supporting mum-to-be with hers is well and good, but have you considered that while the health of your partner and your unborn baby is being checked and re-checked that you too have a 'responsibility' to ensure that yours is up to scratch and lasts long into your greying years of fatherhood? Private health NCTs or 'Wellman' screening tests provide men with the opportunity to have a comprehensive medical check-up.

Dr Tony Foley, a father-of-three and GP in a family practice in Kinsale explains what is involved:

Most checks begin with a lengthy chat with the clinic's doctor. Questions will focus on current medical concerns and broaden to include details on social history: alcohol, cigarettes, work and play.

Family history will be discussed in some detail too. Many common illnesses are strongly familial. Specific male health issues may be explored too.

Next up is the physical exam. This involves blood pressure and pulse check, height, weight and BMI (basal metabolic index – assessment of your ideal weight/height ratio). Heart, lung, abdominal and testicular examinations are performed. For those men over forty-five a rectal examination of the prostate is indicated. A skin or mole-check is worthwhile also. Further examination may be needed if any concerns are raised.

Standard blood tests are then checked, including checks for anaemia, kidney function, liver function, bone profile, cholesterol panel, diabetes, thyroid function, gout and prostate cancer. A heart-tracing (ECG) is performed to look at the electrical activity of the heart and to observe for any rhythm disorders. A urine analysis may diagnose kidney or bladder problems, while an FOB (faecal occult blood) tests for traces of blood in the stool, to screen for bowel cancer. Again, other specific bloods may be requested, depending on relevant medical issues discussed.

Some centres offer optional extras such as hearing tests (audiometry), lung-function tests (spirometry), chest x-ray, cardiac scanning, exercise stress testing, glaucoma screening and bone-density scanning.

The virtues of screening are more easily evident. Earlier diagnosis, timely intervention and appropriate follow-up are all made possible. Convenience, health motivation and adequate time to discuss concerns are all powerful arguments for testing. However, these need to be balanced against potential pitfalls.

The tests are expensive. Costs vary depending on clinic location and services offered. Many GP surgeries offer thorough Wellman checks, while private clinics and hospitals have an extensive selection of investigations. Screening carries the inherent risk of creating and increasing anxiety in the worried-well. False positives can occur, while some tests performed in isolation, or as a snapshot-in-time, are of little clinical value and may be of poor prognostic significance. The focus is on physical health whereas mental health issues and deeper concerns may be overlooked by a physician who is unfamiliar with the patient or his circumstances over time.

We all want that clean bill of health. Our best chance to really achieve that is by eating healthily, exercising frequently and avoiding excessive vices. We should listen intently to our bodies and visit our GPs promptly when the need arises. Health checks are of some value. A healthy lifestyle, however, is priceless.

 WHAT THE EXPERT SAYS: **MIND OVER MUSCLE**

If it's your mission as an expectant dad to get fit for your new family then the first place you must start is with your mind; after all, your mind represents the conception in getting fit. Start with asking yourself:

- What are your habits?
- What do you do on a daily basis that is stopping you from achieving your goals?
- Are you a bad snacker?
- Do you routinely put your workout off as the day goes on and then skip it that night only to tell yourself 'I'll do it tomorrow'?
- What sport or activity would you commit to doing to get fit?
- Can you exercise with your partner?
- Do you love/hate the gym?

Take 15 minutes and write whatever comes to your mind. Don't delete something after you've written it; be honest with yourself. Write down what you want to achieve with your health, including things like how much weight you want to lose or gain, or how much you'd like your waist to shrink by, or even how many push-ups you'd like to be able to do in a minute!

Then write down any obstacles you have in getting fit or maintaining a diet. Once you've written everything out, stand back and take a look at it and see what you can sort out right away and what things can be worked on over time.

Now, pick out a couple of things you can work on within the first two or three weeks, eg sticking to a simple workout, going for a walk/jog twice a week for a half an hour and making sure you eat a healthy breakfast every day. So for the next two weeks, just do that. Then, after those things are habits, pick out a couple more things from your list to work on, eg add a few more exercises to your workout plan, an extra half-hour a week jogging, and concentrate on your diet at mealtimes, including more greens.

This may seem overly simplified, but it works. The reason it works so well is because you're not trying to change everything at once; you're just focusing on a few things at a time. Over the course of the pregnancy, if you do this properly, you should have made a pretty big change to your lifestyle before your new baby arrives. The great part is that it won't feel like a big change because you took 'baby steps', rather than trying to change it all at once.

Ed Scow is a dad-of-two, a personal fitness instructor, author of *The Fit Dad Says* and a regular contributor to *Men's Health*.

The word 'ectopic' means out of place. In this context, it is when the pregnancy develops outside of the uterus (womb). It can occur in several places, but the most common location is within one of the fallopian tubes.

Since an ectopic pregnancy is a potentially life-threatening condition, early diagnosis is essential. The symptoms of an ectopic pregnancy include: severe abdominal pain (low down to one side only), vaginal bleeding or a watery brown discharge, pain in the shoulders, feeling dizzy or faint.

If your partner experiences any of these symptoms she should consult her GP immediately.

The 'M' Word
Miscarriage in pregnancy

If a poll was conducted on what expectant couples think about most during the pregnancy, you can be rest assured that **miscarriage** would be high up on the list. Understandable really, when you consider that 1 in 5 pregnancies in Ireland ends in a miscarriage.

Miscarriages are an unfortunate reality that occurs more commonly within the first trimester of the pregnancy. The vast majority of miscarriages happen early on and are simply bad-luck/chance events. It is important to note that your partner's actions play essentially no role in a miscarriage.

The first sign of a miscarriage may often be your partner feeling something is 'not right'. However, there are physical signs associated with a miscarriage that pregnant women should be on the lookout for, such as vaginal bleeding (particularly if it is prolonged or heavy), weight loss and stomach cramping, as well as contractions.

You should be aware, though, that women can have a spell of bleeding during the early weeks of pregnancy and still go on to have a normal pregnancy. Light bleeding or 'spotting' is common within the first trimester of the pregnancy. However, any bleeding during the pregnancy should always be investigated by contacting your GP, midwife or hospital for immediate advice.

The cause of a miscarriage cannot always be determined. In most cases, the miscarriage occurs because the fertilised egg has not developed properly, or because the baby isn't developing normally. Certain maternal illnesses are associated with an increased risk of miscarriage, although these are very uncommon. Smoking is said to increase the risk of miscarriage, and there is a gradual increase in the risk of miscarriage as a woman gets older.

It is natural to feel loss, sadness, anger, and even guilt, despite the fact that the end result is out of your control. While men do not have to suffer the physical pain associated with a miscarriage they do share the emotional pain of the loss. Women are much more likely to grieve openly and, as a result, are more likely to get support and comfort from friends and family. Men, on the other hand, usually keep their feelings bottled up. You should therefore try to be honest with each other, so that you can each reach a greater understanding of what the other is going through. You should also, at the same time, recognise your partner's need to grieve; affording her time to rest is important as women who have miscarried are likely to feel physically unwell as well as emotionally upset.

There are several organisations that can help with counselling and information on miscarriage, including the Miscarriage Association of Ireland, and The Little Lifetime Foundation (formerly The Irish Stillbirth and Neonatal Death Support Group/ISANDS). You can also ask your GP about miscarriage counselling. If you have been in contact with a hospital during your experience, hospital social workers can also provide counselling.

The majority of couples who have suffered a miscarriage have a high chance of having a healthy baby when they fall pregnant again. How long you wait before deciding whether to get pregnant again is a personal choice. Some couples may wish to try again immediately, while others may prefer to wait.

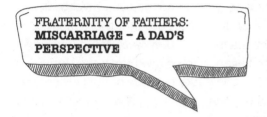

FRATERNITY OF FATHERS:
MISCARRIAGE – A DAD'S PERSPECTIVE

My wife June's first miscarriage was relatively early in pregnancy. And it was just that: 'my wife's miscarriage'. It was all hers. For me, it was a women's medical issue, a gynaecological matter, 'no big deal'. I shrugged it off, concerned only with her healing and getting back to normal. For me, there was no real sense of a loss of a life, just a pregnancy that failed to take off. I don't think that either of us went through a grieving process, certainly I didn't. I just encouraged her to move on and get on with life.

And so we did. As nature took its course, in time June became pregnant again. To be completely honest, I wasn't particularly welcoming of the news. At this point we had two wonderful, healthy children and as far as I was concerned we were complete. But pregnant she was, and so we began to prepare for a new arrival and I started to become more accepting of the situation, even enthusiastic. This time, because of the previous miscarriage, we were more aware of the possibility of things going wrong and had some early scans to see how things were progressing. I clearly remember the last of these scans where we could see the infant's arm apparently waving. Later, we would come to think of this moment as her waving goodbye.

When June told me one day that she hadn't felt any movement for a while, I thought little of it. The earlier movements had been quite faint and surely unborn infants must have quiet periods. But, to reassure her, and encouraged by our GP, we arranged another scan. This time was so different to the earlier ones. When the nurse told me that they could not detect a heartbeat, I simply refused to understand. I thought there must be a problem with the machine, or they were doing it wrong. But no, the truth began to force itself upon me. June was devastated. I felt so guilty because of my earlier lack of enthusiasm about the pregnancy; it was almost like I had put a curse on it.

The next few days are a bit of a blur with some very clear, stark moments remaining etched in my memory. June was admitted a few days later and Julie Ann was delivered at 24 weeks. At this stage, my primary focus was my wife, how to support her, console her and get back to our life together. This was a bit like the first miscarriage but with a bit more fuss and bother.

All of this changed when the nurse asked if we would like to see the baby. June was unsure, but my morbid curiosity impelled me to say 'yes'. And so, little Julie Ann was handed over to us in a kidney bowl, covered in green tissue paper. She was so tiny, yet so perfect. And so, so cold. I wanted to hold her, warm her up and give her the kiss of life. It was all I could do to restrain myself from trying. I had to keep telling myself it was too late; there was nothing I could do.

In an instant, it was no longer just the two of us in the room; now there were three. In that moment, I was transformed from concerned husband to devastated father. Now I suddenly experienced the full reality of what had happened. This was not a women's medical issue; this was a death. My daughter lay dead in my hand, literally.

That was the moment I climbed on board an emotional roller-coaster and strapped myself in for a very rough ride. In the hours and days that followed I experienced emotions I never suspected existed. I went through anger, then resentment, then bitterness, despair and frustration. I cried uncontrollably. Most of all, I felt impotent. I was supposed to be the one to make everything right: the fixer, the protector, the provider. I was failing on all counts and I could do nothing about it.

We buried Julie Ann in the Holy Angels' plot in Glasnevin. As we slowly came to accept what had happened to us, we began to reflect on the first miscarriage and wondered how much we had missed out on. We had never grieved or even really acknowledged our first lost baby. Now we call her Lauren. We don't actually know what sex the baby was, it was too early, but June's instinct tells her it was a girl and that's enough for me.

Julie Ann changed my life. I experienced a whole new set of emotions. It was like going from black and white TV to a full-colour HD screen. Everything was sharper, deeper and richer. The pain was exquisite. But it was not all bad. I learned a new empathy, I became softer, more caring. Some might say I 'got in touch with my feminine side'. It was an experience I would never wish to repeat, but I have grown as a result.

So, there you have it. I cannot speak for all men, just this one man. I suspect most men have a similar experience of miscarriage, some like my first one, a mere medical matter, and some like my second, a death in the family.

Lorcan, Dad of 3, Dublin

'I'm sorry but your baby will most likely not live, there is nothing we can do.'

The medical team were making a fuss of my wife and talking amongst themselves in that hush-hush manner, and then it transpired there was even more bad news to come. She would have to carry the baby to full term, even though there was a chance she, Kate, would not live.

On one of the last visits the senior consultant of the maternity hospital confirmed our little girl had died, and so we decided we wanted our baby delivered there and then, in the hope that we could put this behind us and get on with our lives. However, the new update was my wife had been diagnosed with Grade 5 placenta praevia. I remember thinking it sounded more like Toyota's new range of car. Apparently Grade 5 placenta praevia is the Mercedes of placenta praevia.

The senior consultant was getting nowhere in trying to convince us to wait a little longer, so he left and came back with another doctor.

'Your wife is at risk of dying; however, that is not the biggest risk. If she tries to deliver the baby, she could lose so much blood, she could end up in a vegetative state, but still be alive.'

Fast-forward two months, the saddest funeral I put my family of origin through, and my failure as a father was taking its toll.

Soon afterwards, we found ourselves pregnant again, but sadly this ended in tragedy too. It's classified as a miscarriage, due to weight; however, my son is buried in the same plot as his older sister. The fixer in me decided to research the problem. We got pregnant again very quickly after some of our wounds were licked, but this time we had the research complete. Sure enough, nine months later, we had our second healthy baby. We then presented the research to the hospital as it transpired my wife had some strange blood disorder.

Knowing this and having beaten Fate, I thought I would be free of the guilt and other negative emotions, but this was not the case. It just kept getting worse. Having a healthy child did not negate any loss. We decided we would try one more time and again fell pregnant with ease. We requested the blood-thinning medicine. However, it transpired later, we were prescribed the wrong dose and by 20 weeks our worst fears were realised. We were not going to be taking this baby home either. By this time, my wife had attended counselling. She had encouraged me to do the same, but sure I was ok: why would I need counselling?

Around this time my eldest daughter had a problem with her ear that required some minor surgery; it was also possible that she inherited the same blood-clotting problem. At some point during the testing procedure a doctor from the hospital had to contact me about some aspect of the tests. I gave her a very brief synopsis of what had happened over the years and then she asked me THE QUESTION I had dreaded: HOW ARE YOU?

Sure, I'm grand, not a bother. And that was that!

Truth was I was not grand. A few days later the doctor from the blood clinic called again. She announced that she was not satisfied that I was ok and asked, would I be prepared to see someone?

I attended counselling for ten weeks, working through a lot of issues. Never before would I have been an advocate of counselling but having been knocked down like that, it has helped change my opinion altogether.

We decided not to give in and try just one more time for our last child. Some people, I'm sure, think we were crazy, but we had the knowledge of how to beat this thing and decided to try one last time. Everything was right, and in the end our baby son was born in the summer of 2009.

Given that my wife was strong enough to get through this and keep our family together, it made me realise I was not as strong as I thought, that we all need help when times get hard and more importantly there is nothing to be ashamed of in asking for it.

Colin, Dad of 3, Dublin

For Additional Information log on to:

The Miscarriage Association of Ireland www.miscarriage.ie

A Little Lifetime Foundation (Irish Stillbirth and Neonatal Death Society) www.alittlelifetime.ie

Ectopic Pregnancy Ireland www.ectopicireland.ie

Féileacáin (Stillbirth and Neonatal Death Association of Ireland – SANDAI) www.feileacain.ie

Anam Cara – Supporting Parents after Bereavement www.anamcara.ie

Keeping Mum
The 12-week rule

This is great news, you are a having a baby and family and friends need to be told. But hold on there a minute – or more like 12 weeks, to be precise. With the majority of miscarriages taking place before the twelfth week, many expectant couples decide to postpone the announcement of the pregnancy until reaching this first safety marker or until after the first scan.

Understandably, you are going lady gaga during this period, perhaps paying special attention to expectant work colleagues or friends; you may even be Dan Dare on your lunch hour, surfing for baby names or the latest 'dadgets'. Yet when the time comes to tell all (or a select 'some') you must both be 'universal' in your delivery.

After your respective parents have been informed, close family members should be next on the list. I don't see the lads down the pub being part of this select group, but all families are different!

Though this is indeed great news, try to be sensitive to those who may have been trying to have children themselves for some time or who sadly may have lost a child. Availing of social network sites to inform the masses may not always be the best vehicle for this type of personal news and may be best suited instead for the actual baby announcement.

All in all, only let others know when you are both good and ready to, and tell it in a way that you yourself would like to receive it.

BUMPEDIA: **FLU VACCINE**

Pregnant women are at higher risk of complications from flu, including early labour or severe pneumonia. The risk of these complications is higher after 14 weeks into the pregnancy and is greater for those pregnant women with at-risk medical conditions.

Joe Public v Peter Private
Irish maternity care – an overview

It is at the appointment with her GP to confirm the pregnancy that your partner will receive information on the various choices of maternity care available to her. The main maternity-care options for expectant parents in Ireland are public, semi-private, private and home birth.

Public

◻ Cost: Free

◻ Public patients attend the hospital's antenatal clinic (or hospital clinics based in the community). If your partner's pregnancy is deemed low-risk, she may elect to visit the midwives' clinic, if the hospital has one. This is staffed by experienced midwives and can ensure your continuity of care.

◻ No guarantee mum-to-be will have the same doctor/obstetrician for each antenatal visit.

◻ If it is an uncomplicated birth, a staff midwife, who you may not be familiar with, will deliver your baby.

◻ Following the delivery, your partner will be moved to a public ward where she will stay for up to three days. A small number of hospitals offer an early discharge scheme which allows women to go home early from hospital with follow-up care.

◻ Visiting hours can be restricted as a public patient.

All expectant mothers who are ordinarily resident in the State are entitled to free maternity care regardless of health insurance.

BUMPEDIA: **SHARED CARE**

Shared care (or combined) is when her GP provides about half of the antenatal care with the remaining visits occurring in the maternity hospital. Most GPs are paid by the HSE, so you do not need to pay for any of the visits relating to routine antenatal care and the six-week check-up post partum. Available to public, semi-private and private patients.

Semi-Private

- Cost: Private health insurance usually covers the cost of semi-private accommodation in public hospitals and the cost of delivery; however, you may have to bear the cost of some antenatal visits or scans. Check the details of your health insurance policy to ensure that you are covered and the level of benefit you are entitled to; it would also do no harm to contact your maternity hospital for a list of charges.

- Semi-private care appears to mean different things in different hospitals. If your partner is attending as a semi-private patient, she attends the semi-private clinic. This clinic is run by the consultant and his/her team.

- If it is an uncomplicated birth, a staff midwife, who you may not be familiar with, will deliver your baby.

- Semi-private accommodation can be a 2- or 4-bed room.

Private

- Cost: Private health insurance usually covers the cost of private accommodation in public hospitals and the cost of delivery. Some health insurance companies will pay a contribution to consultant's fees. Check the details of your health insurance policy to ensure that you are covered and the level of benefit you are entitled to and contact your maternity hospital for a list of charges.

- If you are attending privately you will be taken care of by the consultant you have chosen; this also has its benefits, in that you are given a specific date and time for antenatal appointments.

- Your consultant may not necessarily be available to deliver your baby, but there will be a consultant obstetrician on duty who will be in regular contact with your attending midwife for the birth.

- Private care also entitles you to a private room, although, again, this is dependent on availability. Normally, there are no restrictions on visiting times for fathers.

- Private accommodation cannot be booked in advance and is usually allocated on a first-come-first-served basis.

Out on early release

Sounds like criminal terminology, but your partner may be eligible for an **Early Transfer Home**, if she has had a normal birth and has received a full assessment from the medical staff. This means that she can leave the maternity hospital about 12 hours after the birth or, if she gives birth at night, the following day.

I think the phrase 'fair play to them' was coined for these mighty women, and the phrase 'get your skates on' is more appropriate for our new dad who must put the finishing touches to the nursery and get the shopping in!

BUMPEDIA: COMMUNITY AND DOMINO SCHEMES

Often viewed as a compromise between a hospital and home birth, the Domino/Community Midwives schemes allow women who are classified as being low risk (of complications) to see a team of midwives for their antenatal care in the Community/Domino Midwives clinic or in a local health centre free of charge. The Domino service also works in close harmony with general practitioners. The scheme is only available in certain locations throughout Ireland.

With the Community Midwives scheme the birth itself can take place at home, as opposed to the Domino Scheme where the birth takes place in the hospital and mum is discharged several hours afterwards into the care of the midwifery team that cared for her during the pregnancy.

Home birth

In Ireland, any woman who is considered to have a low-risk pregnancy can apply to have a home birth through the director of public health nursing in each HSE area. It is then up to her to source a midwife locally, and that's where the problem lies – there is not a sufficient number of professional midwives who are self-employed to cover the island of Ireland.

According to the latest figures available from the ESRI there is a home birth rate of less than one per cent of all births. However, this small number does not reflect the number of couples who would avail of a home birth if the service was readily available to them. Coincidentally figures from the Home Birth Association of Ireland show that for every woman who gets a planned home birth, there are approximately another ten who would like to have one but who cannot due to lack of service provision.

In certain locations grants are available from the health authorities, but this can vary. If you have private health insurance, a portion of the cost of hiring an independent midwife may be covered.

For many expectant dads, giving birth at home can be a frightening prospect, as if our poor dad-to-be doesn't have enough to worry about. Yet, if you are to look at the big picture, you may find yourself warming up to the idea more than mum herself.

- You can eliminate the stress of breaking down or sitting in rush-hour traffic with a loved one who is well on her journey to giving birth.

- You are more relaxed and in control in your own surroundings.

- You can draw on family or close friends for their support.

- There is no going home alone after your baby is born.

- There are no unfamiliar faces, medical equipment or other expectant mums giving birth in your living room.

- You can set your own visiting times.

- If there are other siblings in the home, a home birth provides an opportunity for all the family to get involved so no one is left out. It can also create an immediate bond between siblings.

- But most importantly, you can have as much tea and toast as you like.

Sound's great – so where do we sign up? As with all things in life, especially new life, there are factors to consider:

Risk: Your partner must be seen to be in a low-risk category first by her GP and an independent midwife.

Location: In the event that there are complications with the birth and your partner must be moved to hospital, you must consider your proximity to the hospital or the speed in which emergency services can reach your location.

Space: Can your home accommodate a birthing pool and all of its contents?

Drugs (for her, you dummy!): Unless you plan on hiring your very own anaesthetist then an epidural is out of the question.

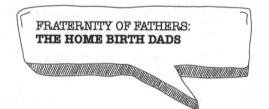

FRATERNITY OF FATHERS:
THE HOME BIRTH DADS

The birth was going to happen within an hour or two, so we moved into the living room – the cosiest room in our house – with the lights off, and I sat in a chair, supporting my wife's crouched body as she rocked back and forth. Keeping her hair back, offering her water, whispering words of encouragement, all helped her through the final stages of this labour. When the baby arrived the midwife handed him to me immediately. It was amazing to hold him in my arms as the midwife looked after my wife.

At home with my family, my friends and my new son, I relaxed in our living room, eating toast, drinking tea and sipping champagne. After a while, we headed up to bed with our baby and cuddled in beside our sleeping daughter. The following morning she woke to discover her new brother and leaned over to kiss him.

David, Dad of 2, Cork

When my wife broached the notion of a home birth I was a little reluctant especially as this was our first baby. I always felt that hospitals were the safest place to have a baby, in case something was to go wrong. My wife was adamant though and made a drive at getting as much information for us on the subject as possible. You can sit back a little when it's a hospital birth, but when it's taking place in your own home, you seem to take on a greater responsibility in getting involved with the whole thing.

Our midwife was excellent; she became more of a family friend really. My wife's sister and our two mums were also there for the delivery. My wife used a birthing pool and I helped support her with her breathing, changing the music and making the odd cup of tea. It was all very relaxed, and when our son was born it was really special to be able to hold him for the very first time in our own living room.

Tomas, Dad of 1, Sligo

I don't know how many times I said 'are you sure?', 'you won't be able to call out for an epidural if you cannot stand the pain', but at the end of the day it's what my wife wanted. Now having gone through it twice I can understand why my wife felt so strongly about it; it's not as if we are any sort of new-age family, far from it, in fact, but it was right for us and while I accept that there is uncertainty with everything in life, thankfully there were no complications with both births and we were able to enjoy the experience to the fullest.

Geoff, Dad of 2, Galway

It's not for everyone, I admit, and being the most nervous man on the planet, I was not happy with the idea at all and did try my utmost to change my partner's mind on numerous occasions, in fact. I did play the 'but it's my baby too and what if something happens' card. I decided to school myself and watch a few DVDs on home-birthing (and I'm squeamish) and even though I expected to be horrified, I wasn't – not really. By talking to other parents I changed my opinion and was actually more in favour of it than my wife was. Birthing at home has been around for thousands of years; it is not a new phenomenon. As an expectant dad you will feel very anxious, but if you surround yourself with professionals and you get informed, then you will feel a whole lot better about the situation.

John, Dad of 1, Dublin

For additional information log on to:

Cuidiu – The Irish Childbirth Trust www.cuidiu-ict.ie

Citizens Information www.citizensinformation.ie

Association for Improvements in the Maternity Services www.aimsireland.com

Home Birth Association of Ireland www.homebirth.ie

Testing, Testing ...
Scans and checks

The scan for the majority of expectant fathers is like wining the lotto – you cannot really believe it's happening until you are holding the proof in your hand. And that proof comes in the form of the first picture. The first picture is the final strike three for dads-to-be. We've had the positive pee-stick, the GP nod and now here you are staring up at a small blob which confirms that you are about to embark on one of my most exciting journeys of your life – that of fatherhood.

BUMPEDIA: **THE ULTRASOUND**

An essential tool in ensuring that your baby is growing and developing normally, ultrasound scans have been in existence for nearly fifty years.

Ultrasound pictures are created by using sound waves. First a gel is applied to your partner's belly, and then a small hand-held device (a transducer) is moved over her skin, which sends sound waves through her body that reflect off her internal organs creating an image. An ultrasound scan is a painless procedure which takes between 10 and 15 minutes and is carried out by a sonographer or consultant.

Work it out

If you have arranged to attend appointments during the working day, be prepared that seldom are they on time, therefore do not commit yourself to returning to the workplace at a particular time. There is, however, a provision in place that gives you paid time off from work to attend the two antenatal classes preceding the birth (see the section on antenatal classes in Chapter 3).

The number of scans available to your partner will be dependent on what maternity hospital she is attending and whether she is a public or private patient. The **Dating Scan** (in or around the 12-week mark) and the **Anomaly Scan** (around the 20-week mark) are considered by many fathers as the two most important scans that expectant dads should make every effort to attend.

As the name suggests, the **Dating Scan** gives a more accurate **Expected Date of Delivery** (EDD). It can also tell if there is more than one baby, how your baby is developing and if there are any signs of abnormalities.

If the dating scan is the first look-see for expectant fathers, then expect to be blown away by the **Anomaly Scan.**

What's up, Doc?
Monitoring mum

At various stages throughout the pregnancy your partner's health will be monitored. Aside from weight screening, blood pressure, urine and blood tests, there are circumstances where additional tests may be required. This may be the case if your partner is a certain age, has a particular medical history or suffers from a genetic condition, and there are concerns surrounding the possibility of giving birth to an infant with a chromosome problem, eg Down Syndrome.

The **Panorama Test** analyses cell-free DNA circulating in the pregnant mother's blood. It is a new option in prenatal screening for chromosome syndromes. This test can be requested for any single pregnancy. The appointment will include a blood test and an ultrasound scan to confirm dates and viability.

The **Harmony Test** is a new option in prenatal screening for Down Syndrome and other foetal chromosomal conditions. This test can be requested for any pregnancy from 10 weeks, including in vitro fertilization (IVF) pregnancies with egg donors. It can also be requested for twin pregnancies conceived naturally or by IVF using the patient's own egg.

A **nuchal scan** is when an ultrasound is taken to measure the translucent area in the skin on the back of the baby's neck (the nuchal fold), to determine whether there is a risk of the baby developing a chromosomal abnormality, such as Down Syndrome. If the results show that your partner is in the high-risk category, she may be advised to have the following tests:

Chorionic villus sampling (CVS) involves taking a sample of some of the placental tissue to check for any genetic abnormalities in the pregnancy, such as Down Syndrome or Cystic Fibrosis.

Similar to CVS, **amniocentesis** is where a needle is passed into a pregnant woman's womb and some fluid is removed from around the baby. CVS is normally carried out during the first trimester, between weeks 10 and 13 of the pregnancy, while amniocentesis is carried out at a later stage, between weeks 15 and 20. Apart from the discomfort associated with these tests, there is also a small risk of miscarriage. These tests can also cause distress for expectant parents as results are not immediate and may involve going private.

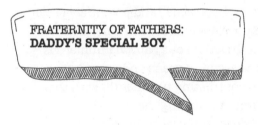

FRATERNITY OF FATHERS:
DADDY'S SPECIAL BOY

'The news isn't good. Your baby has Down Syndrome. I am sorry.'

Having heard the above, whilst cocooned with the wife in our car on a drab, grey Dublin street just over one year ago, I would never have imagined I would find myself where I am today. We had waited a week from the time of the amniocentesis test to that phone call, and to finally hear the confirmation from the doctor on the phone, set in motion a series of life-changing decisions and realities. The news the doctor had given us was something we had only recently been asked to consider, but here we were now, locked in our car, as the grey streets around us reflected our souls at that moment, desperately looking for some direction or approval that we were going to be ok, faced with the life-altering news that our unborn baby had Down Syndrome.

So, my baby has Down Syndrome. What is this and what does it mean? To the layman, as I most certainly was at that time, Down Syndrome is an intellectual disability, caused by a triplication of the number 21 chromosome, affecting, on average, about 1 in 800 babies in Ireland. As we were reliably informed by the various doctors throughout the pregnancy, by deciding to continue with the pregnancy (tragically we were given that predicament to consider) our baby could hope to achieve the mental capabilities of a 12–13-year-old child and then remain at that stratum for the remainder of their life, which incidentally would also not be as long as a 'normal' person. We were told to expect heart conditions, poor eyesight, poor hearing, low muscle tone (known as 'hypotonia') and potential speech and language difficulties. We absorbed this news as we steadily followed the growth of our baby via numerous ultrasound scans, the seeming peace and serenity the baby was existing in contrasting turbulently with the chaos around our own lives during that time.

Attempting to come to terms with this news was unlike anything I have ever experienced. I had no semblance of a precedent to draw on, extremely limited experience of any kind of disabilities or special needs, and on a more basic level, I was still coming to terms with the fact that I was going to be a Daddy, let alone a 'special needs Daddy', whatever that may entail. Myself and the wife got in touch with Down Syndrome Ireland and the Down Syndrome Dublin branch and through this organisation we arranged to meet with a counsellor to try and make some sense of the situation we were thrust into. This was of enormous help to both of us. We were given the reassurance we needed to grieve the life we thought we were going to have and we were helped take the first steps towards the new path laid out before us. We spent countless hours scouring the web for information, often delighting in the glorious stories and pictures we came across, but equally finding ourselves faced with negative stories, opinion and experiences that scared us violently to our very core. The blessed curse of the web in stark reality!

Since our baby boy, Noah, was born we have had numerous appointments to fulfil in various hospitals and clinics across Dublin. He has been in Our Lady's Children's Hospital, Crumlin, for heart exams, hearing exams and eyesight exams. He has physiotherapist and speech and language therapist visits from St Michael's House, his service provider, and also still attends the baby clinic at the Coombe Women's Hospital, where he first made an entrance into our lives. Thankfully, his legion of appointments have not turned up anything too dramatic; he has three small 'manageable' holes in his heart, potentially a slight hearing deficiency in his left ear and great eyesight as things stand. His physiotherapy is progressing well, to the point he can now stand upright whilst holding onto the sofa and we are incessantly trying to get him to utter his first 'Dada' or 'Mama', to no avail so far, but we plough on regardless.

Noah is now eight months old and I wouldn't trade him, or any of his 'specialness', for all the sand in Egypt. He is a most delightful little boy and regularly now happily sits upright on his play mat, playing and jabbering away with his toys and has already established a gang of friends thanks to Mummy's weekly tea and cake group. To be told at the very start of this adventure by a doctor that he was sorry for me almost makes me laugh now when I think about it, because the truth is I am the one who is now sorry, sorry for everyone who cannot see Noah and share in his and our lives. That is the only thing about Down Syndrome that warrants any sorrow, and I for one am delighted that I have reached this reality now.

Martin, Dad of 2, Dublin

For additional information log on to:

Down Syndrome Ireland www.downsyndrome.ie

Down Syndrome Dublin www.dsdublin.ie

St Michael's House www.smh.ie

Our Lady's Children's Hospital, Crumlin www.olchc.ie

BUMPEDIA: **WHAT IS RHESUS NEGATIVE?**

Everybody's blood is either rhesus positive or rhesus negative, regardless of your blood group. The majority of people have rhesus positive (Rh+) blood cells but about 15 per cent of people have rhesus negative (Rh-).

If mum-to-be is rhesus negative and your baby happens to be positive (usually your baby's blood type will not be known until the delivery), this can cause problems. If your partner's blood comes into contact with your baby's blood, eg if your partner has an accident, her antibodies can attack your baby's rhesus positive blood cells. Although low levels of antibodies won't usually cause harm to your baby, high levels can cause problems.

During early antenatal appointments your partner will be given a series of blood tests, one of which will determine whether she is rhesus negative. If she is, she will be continually checked during her pregnancy for any signs of antibodies.

If your partner gives birth to a baby with rhesus positive blood, there is a risk of Rh antibodies developing causing a haemolytic disease of the newborn in a future pregnancy. Anti-D is given to the mother within 72 hours of birth, or miscarriage, as an injection to prevent this happening.

Join the Club
The waiting room

Though being present at the scan is very important, the build-up to seeing your heir in black and white can be an anxious time for many expectant dads, especially as there is a degree of waiting involved (which is understandable when you consider that you are in a maternity hospital and babies are being born, so in their defence the wonderful midwives and obstetricians may be otherwise engaged). This is why the game of people-watching was invented in a hospital waiting room, no more so than in your local maternity hospital or clinic. To pass the time, figure out which member of the expectant dads club you belong to:

The Shuffler: You know the guy – the one who cannot sit still, keeps looking at his watch whilst tapping the appointment card and throwing his eyes to the heavens. He's been out twice already to glare at the receptionist and is now off to check the parking meter even though he's only been in the room for ten minutes.

The Tycoon: That's him over there with his copy of *Wired*. Between breaks in reading he can be heard quite loudly saying to his wife, 'I have to take this call, it's important.' No doubt he's on first names with the staff, having never met them before.

The Sleeper: Head back, mouth wide open, this fella is glad of the rest.

The Talker: Happy to chat away with anybody who will listen, especially the expectant mums. You could put it down to nerves, but his partner's painful grin tells us that he's like this all the time.

The Breeder: Arrives at the appointment with all his kids in tow, followed by a very worn-out 'been-here, done-it-all-before' mum-to-be. Any new expectant dad who witnesses the spectacle of crying, crisp-eating, scrapping monkeys in the centre of the floor may be forgiven for thinking, 'What have I got myself in for?' Rest assured, it's in the rearing!

The Quarterback: Sits on the edge of his chair with his legs wide open, furiously texting on his mobile phone – how many mates does this guy have! If that's not enough, his spontaneous fits of laughter seem to drown out that exact moment that the next patient is called.

The Honeymooner: We can tolerate everyone else, but if there is one dad-to-be that we all share a universal dislike for, it's this guy. We can hear him before we see him: 'Slowly now, hun.' He enters the waiting room at a snail's pace, clutching his partner's upper arm. When he finally lands down in his seat beside his partner he caresses her bump-less belly and leans in to her, whispering sweet nothings that evoke a giddy teenage response. When her name is called we endure the spectacle in reverse, but are pleased to see him leave – that is, until we realise that this same guy is going to ask a lot of questions, and I mean *a lot* of questions.

Tips on attending the scan

- Check the parking situation and ensure you have sufficient change for the meter, or sign up for ParkingTag if it's available in your area.

- If you are unable to attend appointments, organise for a relative or close friend (hers, not yours!) to go instead.

- Bring along some reading material, in the event that you are not seen on time.

- Keep two multigrain bars in her handbag in case you both get the nibbles.

- Get out of the corner – you haven't been grounded; position yourself so you can see what's going on.

- There may be silences as the sonographer or consultant goes about their business so don't go guessing that this means something is wrong.

- When your partner is having her ultrasound don't be afraid to ask questions, no matter how foolish you think they are.

- Assist your partner with her personal items; after all, no one can see you holding a handbag in a darkened room.
- Don't forget the picture!

Picture this

The picture of your unborn baby is the ultimate prize from your visit. But be warned, ultrasound pictures are printed using thermal imaging paper which can turn brown when exposed to light and heat.

Laminating would seem like an obvious tool for preserving your treasured picture; however, the process works in the opposite way, by destroying the image due to the level of heat that is emitted. Similarly photocopying should also be avoided. A safer option is to scan the image onto your PC, up to the cloud or simply snap a shot on your phone to share with family & friends. If you hanker after a wallet keepsake that you can proudly show off to family and friends, or if doting grandparents-to-be would be delighted to have their own copies, then print out the image onto photo paper.

BUMPEDIA: **CROWN TO RUMP**

The term 'from crown to rump' refers to your baby being measured from the top of its head to its bottom, as opposed to 'from head to toe', as the legs are curled up to the baby's stomach.

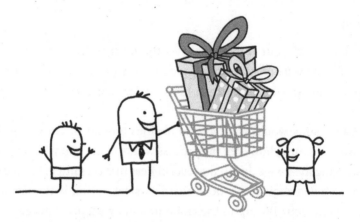

'A father carries pictures where his money used to be.'

Author Unknown

2 The Second Trimester
When reality 'kicks' in

Trimester 2: Weeks 13-28

For many expectant mums (and dads) the second trimester provides a very welcome respite from the early pregnancy symptoms suffered in the first trimester. A 'real' connection exists, with many women saying that they begin to 'feel' pregnant during this period. Expectant fathers see their partners beginning to show more, and they can begin to develop a bond with the unborn baby, especially when they feel the baby kicking later on, or when they see them close up at the ultrasound scan.

When you reach the second trimester you can start telling family and close friends the good news, decide if you wish to know the sex of the baby, debate over baby names and feel a little more at ease since the risk of miscarriage is much lower once you have seen through the first trimester.

Womb with a view

The second trimester is when your baby really comes into her own, literally speaking, as she begins to resemble a newborn with distinguishable human features. Organs develop further and start functioning and muscles grow stronger and your baby begins to store up fat. She will also be putting on weight at about 100g (3.5oz) per week. Meconium grows in your baby's intestinal tract which ends up being your baby's first bowel movement. If you are having a boy, the testes are descending from the abdomen; in girls, the uterus and ovaries are in place.

In the final few weeks of the second trimester the body is almost fully formed and more proportionate; however, the lungs are not quite developed and will not be for some time. If your baby was to be delivered now, she may survive with the assistance of medical care.

Baby talk

'You'd better not be serious about any funny baby names because not only can I hear you, I can also give as good a kick as Bruce Lee. I can open my eyes but I can't see anything yet, even though my eyelashes and eyebrows are growing. My fingernails continue to grow, which is handy in case I have an itch, but fear not, my wrinkly red skin is protected by a fine hair called "lanugo" and a waxy protective coating called "vernix". By the end of the second trimester, I am about 12in long (30.5cm) and weigh about 2lbs (0.91kg).'

Mum's the word

Undoubtedly, one of the biggest milestones in the second trimester will be the moment your partner experiences her first 'flutter' – when the baby moves for the first time. For most women it occurs between the 18th and 20th week of the pregnancy and tends to be earlier for women expecting their second or subsequent babies. As the months progress, she will experience some weight gain and her abdomen will begin to expand to accommodate a growing baby, and she may need to start wearing maternity clothes.

She'll more than likely still be suffering from varying emotions (mood swings!) due to the changes that are taking place to her body so 'sensitivity' and 'support' should be two of the most frequently used words in the expectant dad's dictionary during this trimester.

Symptom sympathy

While your partner may no longer be suffering from morning sickness or nausea, and may have more energy, there are other symptoms of the pregnancy that are common in the second trimester, including heartburn and indigestion, constipation, varicose veins, haemorrhoids and aches and pains in her abdomen, groin, thighs or back. For many women stretch marks will start to show up on their bellies, legs and breasts – most of which will fade after childbirth.

The second trimester is often referred to as the 'golden trimester' of the pregnancy and your partner may begin to 'glow'. Fear not, we are not talking about some florescent-painted exterior but a healthy glowing appearance, attributed to a reduction in first trimester symptoms, an increased circulation to meet baby's needs and a general all-round sense of well-being that does not entail sprinting to the loo. If your partner complains of lacking illumination – probably because you forgot to mention it, you dummy – it's most likely that you are expecting a boy. Well, that's what 'they' say – glow for a girl, no glow for a boy.

This is not a 'golden' opportunity for any dad-to-be to think he has his partner back to full capability for a few months. All pregnancies are different. Your partner may no longer be reaching for the basin to catch her morning vomit, but she still has a tiny being growing inside of her who may have her own ideas on how she is feeling on a daily basis.

Kicking in

The realisation that you are to be a dad will start to sink in in the 'middle months', and it is only natural to have concerns of your own regarding what type of father you will be and the financial worries that having children entails. The second trimester opens the door for expectant dads to become more involved in the pregnancy. Now that your baby is able to hear what is going on outside, expectant dads can seize on this opportunity to bond with their unborn baby. The first time you feel the kick (or punch!) will be a 'wow' moment for you. It is also a period when dad-to-be can see baby up close during the antenatal visit. It may not be possible for you to attend all of the antenatal visits with your partner, but you should do your best to attend the appointments where the main ultrasound scans are performed, especially if want to share in knowing the sex of your baby.

Congratulations, you are halfway there.

In My Day ...
Handling advice

Oh yes, once the cat is out of the bag, the flood gates will truly open and out will flow a tsunami of advice, tips, and tricks on surviving the pregnancy and the early stages of parenting.

It may feel as if nothing else is going on in your life with sisters, mothers, work colleagues asking you for a full run-down on how mum-to-be is doing. You will feel sidelined, and tempted as you may be to say 'what about me?', try to hold back; your consolation and support network will come in the form of your fellow man. He will politely enquire as to your choice of baby names, express serious interest when it comes to the latest baby gadget, and he will hug you so tightly as if it's your last goodbye and whisper 'watch out for the sleep, watch out for the sleep ...'

Take all advice with a pinch of salt; it is with good intention after all. Pay special attention to any family members or friends who have more than the one child as they are best placed to tell you what mistakes they made with their first and what they did differently next time round.

BUMPEDIA: **CARPAL TUNNEL SYNDROME (CTS)**

Within the wrist, nerves and tendons pass through a space called the carpal tunnel. As the carpal tunnel is somewhat narrow, a major nerve (the median) that passes through this tight space can become irritated or compressed, resulting in pain, numbness and a burning or tingling sensation in the hand and fingers.

Women are three times more likely than men to develop carpal tunnel syndrome, and 50 per cent of pregnant women suffer from CTS in the later stage of their pregnancy. Treatment consists of wrist splints, anti-inflammatory medication and cortisone injections which can all help contribute to reducing swelling. However, CTS in pregnant women often improves within the first few months of the baby being born. There have been also reported cases of new dads suffering from CTS, but this is due to holding or feeding your newborn incorrectly!

Nobody Puts Baby in a Corner!
Preparing a child for the new arrival

In the 'who-do-we-tell' list, expectant parents can often neglect to include those closest to them who will be most affected by the new addition – their children. The age of your child (or children) will be a factor in how the news is received, with excitement and curiosity being at the forefront of emotional responses. Of course, there will be more important questions requiring delicate answers: 'How did he get in there in the first place?' And better yet, 'How does he get out of there?'

Being the number one in your parents' eyes is a mantle no young child will be willing to let go of too easily. They will treat any obstacle with great suspicion. After all, Daddy's little princess or toy soldier has been used to having his/her way this entire time, along with all the toys! The concept of sharing (of any kind) will be alien to him, and going from the undivided to the divided can be a daunting experience for any child.

The key to a successful transition is to involve your child in the pregnancy from the very moment you tell them the news. The following tips will help you in preparing your child for the new arrival:

Lead by example: Organise play dates with friends which involves two siblings from the one family, especially if one is a baby. This way you can show your child the advantages of having a baby sister or brother within the family.

Name calling: Allow your child to suggest names for the baby, though best of luck explaining why Spiderman or Peppa may not be a suitable name to go along with Murphy!

Bump brothers: Allow him to rub/listen to the bump like Daddy does.

Present a 'present': Let him pick out a present for the new baby that he can keep safe until the new arrival comes home. At this stage, it is also a good idea to consider buying a present **from** your new baby to be given to the new brother or sister when they first meet.

'Bigger' not older: Remind him that he will be a 'bigger' brother/sister and that his job as 'the bigger one' is to look after his 'little' brother/sister.

Role play: A baby doll is a useful tool to demonstrate to your child what it can be like to have a baby in the home, though don't be horrified if the doll goes missing only to be found in next door's dog kennel!

Post fall-out: When siblings meet the new addition for the first time, pay special attention that no child is left out or ignored by parents or relatives. If your child wants to hold the baby, don't be quick to disregard their request as this is a great way for siblings to become acquainted; instead sit down beside them and help them to cradle the baby. Great chance for the new family photo!

iDad: **ALL HANDS ON DECK**

Expectant dads should take up the slack when it comes to telling their offspring why mum needs to rest or is unable to engage in activities that she was used to doing prior to the pregnancy. Dad-to-be should also create fun ways for the rest of the family to help mum-to-be during the pregnancy, eg preparing a special breakfast, organising a surprise outing or making a card for mum-to-be with the whole family wishing her well.

Woof Time of It
Your dog and your unborn baby

Preparing the family dog for the arrival of a new baby can begin early on in the pregnancy.

- Don't wait until the very last minute to put all the baby equipment in position. This will only confuse your dog, making him/her anxious about a new change that may be taking place in the household. The sooner your pet becomes familiar with the new items, the more at ease he/she will be when your baby comes home.

- In the same manner as you would prepare a child, demonstrate what will happen by using a doll to change or bathe.

- Brush up on any dog commands that you may find useful when baby is home and ensure that all his/her vaccinations are up-to-date.

- There are recordings available of baby sounds that can be played to your pet so that they can become accustomed to any new noises that may come from your baby.

NEVER leave a pet alone with a baby.

iDad: PREGNANCY MOVIES FOR MEN

Due Date – to know what it's really like when your partner goes into labour and you are some distance away with an AH for company.

Children of Men – shows you how protective you can be over a pregnant woman. You're played by Clive Owen – yeah of course you are, I suppose it's better than being Hugh Grant ...

Nine Months – when you don't take the news of the pregnancy too well, especially seeing as you have to wave goodbye to your cat and Porsche, but you come good in the end (the very 'very' end!).

Father of the Bride 2 – if a movie can have too many pregnancy hormones bounding about all at once, then this is it. You sell your house, you buy it back for more, you have to organise a baby shower and manage an annoying French dude called Franc.

Knocked Up – after a one-night-stand ends with herself getting pregnant, you're not so sure if you are ready for fatherhood and you're not too ashamed to let her know it either.

Junior – when the shoe is on the other foot and you want to try the pregnancy on for size!

Lethal Weapon 4 – now we are talking, something for everyone: gun fights, unusual cravings, car chases and waters breaking.

Boss Baby – essentially illustrates who's really in charge once you have a baby (you guessed it: the baby). The inimitable Alec Baldwin, who voices the mini boss, is reason enough to watch.

I Can't See Him as a Thor FitzGerald!
The baby name game

10 rules for choosing a name

1. Be diplomatic: Don't go all gung-ho with the 'well, if it's a boy he has to be called ...' attitude. Instead, get out two sheets of paper and each write down your top five boy and girl names, then swop them over and rank one another's from 1–5 in order of preference. Remember, compromise is another way of saying 'that'll do as a middle name'. Better yet ask the bump, a kick is a yes and no activity means he's asleep!

2. Say the name out in different tones, eg

Happy – as if he has just taken his first steps.

Outrage – when he decides to smear his nappy across the widescreen TV.

Sadness – when he decides to go backpacking for a year and you'll miss him greatly (trust me you will!).

3. Can the name be **shortened**, and if so are you satisfied with the result – and more importantly, will baby Jim Bob be?

4. Are there any obvious **nicknames** that your child may end up having to live with? Be sure to check that the **initials** work with the surname and don't spell out anything which may draw unnecessary schoolyard attention, eg **V**ictor **D**'Arcy. Although toss in a middle name or a double-barrelled alternative and it paints a completely different picture, eg **V**incent **I**an **P**urcell.

5. A class act: There is nothing more heart-wrenching than hearing your littlest one say, 'Daddy you said I was special but there are five Bellas in my class.' Will you mind your child sharing the same name as others in her class? Similarly be fair to the wee lad or lass when it comes to spelling and pronunciation; we all know it's great to be different but think about the first-day-of-school-sticker scenario!

6. Brittany and Brad: If you are to amble down the road of celebrity names, be conscious of the fact that celebrities tend to lead different lives to us mortals, so today's tabloid angel could be tomorrow's devil.

7. They grow up so fast: What's cute for the first 16 years of their lives may not be so convincing when they are negotiating a deal-breaker in the boardroom later in adult life.

8. Adolf means 'noble wolf': Look at the meaning of your baby's name. You don't want to find out afterwards that your chosen name translates as 'unmanly' or worse still, that your little girl's name means 'the chaser of men'.

9. Keep it in the family: A neutral option would be to decide if it's a boy then the father's (or his father's etc) name is chosen; if it's a girl then it'll be the mother's (or her mother's etc) name. With regard to subsequent children, just reverse the principle, and I don't mean if it's a boy then it's the mother's name!

10. First impressions may change everything: You may be both adamant on the name, but what can occur is when you are cradling your newborn for the very first time you suddenly look down and realise that he or she doesn't look at all like an Ethan or an Isabel for that matter. Don't panic, time is very much on your side as you have up to 12 weeks to register the name after your baby is born.

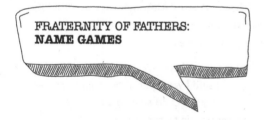

FRATERNITY OF FATHERS:
NAME GAMES

My pal was picking up his daughter from playschool when he heard a staff member telling a 'Pocahontas' and a 'Princess' to stop pulling 'Dora's' hair. Surely they were role playing, weren't they?

Martin, Dad of 3, Meath

The results are in ...

The CSO released its statistics on Irish baby names in 2017, with Jack and Emily taking top spot for most popular names last year.

The top five names for boys were Jack, James, Daniel, Conor and Sean, while the top five for girls were Emily, Emma, Amelia, Grace and Sophie.

New names in the top 100 for last year are Theo and Jackson for boys, and Aoibhin, Nina, Pippa and Esma for girls.

There was more variety in names for girls than boys, with 4,493 girls' names registered compared to 3,472 boys' names.

Battle of the sexes: gender selection

Ultimately the gender of your baby is determined by the combination of two sex chromosomes. Your partner's egg contains an X chromosome whilst your sperm contributes a 'deciding' Y or X chromosome. Should your sperm contain an X chromosome then you are having a girl, a Y means a boy. Speculation on gender selection will also depend on the different characteristics of the sperm – the speed, survival rate in the womb and which type of sperm can withstand the different pH-levels (acidity) in the vagina.

It is normal practice for every expectant parent to secretly root for team blue or team pink. However, we are universal as expectant parents that a healthy baby will always take precedence over the sex. And anyway, who said daddy's little princess couldn't play ball?

Is That His Little ...?
Finding out the sex of your baby

The **20-week scan** or anomaly scan plays an important part in the pregnancy as it provides an opportunity for expectant parents to get a better picture (literally) on how their baby is developing, and for the sonographer or obstetrician to determine if any abnormalities exist. Your baby's overall health and growth is assessed, and limbs, organs, heart, spine, head and the position of the placenta and the fluid that surrounds your baby will also be checked. It is at the 20-week scan that expectant parents can also first discover the sex of the baby (or babies!).

Right up to the very moment that the jelly is applied to the bump couples have been divided on whether to find out the sex of their baby or to hold off until the main event.

Of course finding out can be very exciting. Expectant parents can often feel a closer bond to their unborn baby now that they are aware of its gender; the 'is it a he or a she' factor is whittled down to leave just the one finalist. In the journey home afterwards baby names are automatically eliminated and the warring factions of team pink and team blue now have a champion. Though there has to be a 'loser', consider this, there's always next time ...

Old-wife methods of determining the sex of your baby

1. **One ring to rule**: Suspend a ring on a piece of string over your partner's belly. If the ring swings back and forth, it's a girl. If it swings in a circle then it's a boy.

2. **Take a walk on the 'wide' side**: If your partner is carrying all the baby weight out front, it's a boy; if she puts on extra weight around her hips and bum and generally has a wide bump, then it's a girl.

3. **The answer is down the loo**: Severe morning sickness is often an indicator that you are having a girl.

4. Beat this: If your baby's heartbeat is above 140 then you are having a girl, and if it is below 140 then you are having a boy.

5. The 'breast' way: If your partner's left breast is bigger than the right breast – during pregnancy, I might add – it's a girl; if the right breast is bigger, then it's a boy.

WHAT THE EXPERT SAYS: 3D/4D SCANS

One of the most popular pregnancy scans in Ireland today is the 3D/4D scan. A 3D ultrasound uses hundreds of pictures of your baby to produce a 3D high-resolution image, while a 4D ultrasound takes the 3D scan images and adds the element of time to the process, streaming it into a live-action animated DVD of your baby.

A 3D/4D scan uses the same sound frequency as a normal 2D black-and-white scan and is considered extremely safe for mother and baby. There is no need for a doctor's referral letter; however, this scan does not replace a complete diagnostic ultrasound scan with your own midwife/obstetrician or maternity hospital.

There is no problem performing the 3D/4D scan at any time during the pregnancy, but in the earlier stages of pregnancy, the baby is sometimes too small in the images to benefit from 3D/4D ultrasound, so most ultrasound clinics will perform the scan from 22 weeks until 33 or 34 weeks, the optimum time being between 24 and 29 weeks of pregnancy.

Sometimes it may happen that baby has his/her hands in front of the face and/or the legs are in the way, which will make it difficult to get good quality pictures. If this happens, your partner may be asked to take a walk and a fizzy drink to get baby moving around to obtain better pictures. If mum-to-be is diabetic or glucose intolerant, an ice-cold drink of water should often do the trick.

The 3D/4D scan usually takes half an hour and clients receive at least four colour 3D prints, between ten and twenty colour 3D pictures on a CD that you can print and email, and at least two black-and-white 2D prints. A DVD is also taken of any movement the baby makes and is normally about 20–25 minutes long. You can also find out the sex of the baby, if you wish, but there is no problem if you want to keep the gender a mystery!

Paula Tunney DCR (D) DML founder of of BabyScan

Seeing Things
Expecting multiples

Finding out at your first scan that you are expecting twins (or more!) can come as a quite a shock to many expectant parents – even for those undergoing fertility treatment, such as IVF, which is more likely to produce a multiple pregnancy than a natural conception.

The shock will not last for very long, and excitement and getting on with the job at hand will take over. From here on in, your head will condition itself to thinking in two's, though it will hurt somewhat from the associated outlay that comes with having twins – double the nappies, the clothes, the pram, the cots, the bottles, the education ... I'll stop there!

It is important to note that extra care should be taken with regard to a multiple pregnancy as there is a risk of complications including miscarriage, pre-term birth, and low birthweight. It should come as no surprise that your partner will be wearier from carrying two or more down front, and as an expectant dad of multiples you will need to show her a great deal of support especially in the final stages of the pregnancy.

Expectant parents of multiples are advised to get in touch with **The Irish Multiple Births Association (IMBA). The IMBA** is a charitable organisation run by volunteers who are all parents of multiples themselves and who offer a unique insight into the issues facing expectant parents and families of multiples during pregnancy, birth and the different stages of childhood.

 For additional information log on to:
www.imba.ie

In the company of men — Famous dads of twins

Robert De Niro
Al Pacino
Charlie Sheen
Mel Gibson
Denzel Washington
Chris 'Thor' Hemsworth
Jay-Z
Cristiano Ronaldo
George Clooney

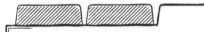

BUMPEDIA: TWIN-to-TWIN TRANSFUSION SYNDROME

A disease of identical twin foetuses caused by abnormal connecting blood vessels in the twins' placenta, resulting in an imbalanced flow of blood from one twin to another. In other words, the placenta gives more blood and nutrients to one twin while starving the other, which can be very serious for the survival and health of both twins.

When I discovered we were going to be parents of twins,
I was working in Rathcoole, Dublin, as a plasterer. We
were doing an office inside a warehouse. My partner
phoned me as she had just come out of Holles Street
and said could I talk for a minute, I said ok and she
asked where I was. I told her I was up a scaffolding doing
taping and jointing. She asked me to get down and I
suspected the worse. So I went outside and she told me
I was going to be the daddy of twins. My heart sank and
I felt a cold fear go through me. It wasn't that I didn't
want them; it was the fact that I was afraid of being a
dad to one, let alone two. I just wasn't sure if I could be
a good dad as it was all new to me. The phone call was
quite short as my partner said, 'I'll let it sink in and talk
to you later.' I went back to work and wasn't my usual
happy self. I was worried. Could I handle this? I swore
continually for about forty-five minutes which is kind
of accepted on a building site and eventually one of the
lads said, 'You ok?' I told him what had happened and
he said, 'Oh Horlicks', or words to that effect. We went for
coffee because work was the last thing on my mind and
when it sank in, it was calming delight.

Ian, Dad of 2, Dublin

On 1 December 2010, my wife Mandy and I were blessed
by the arrival of our 8 weeks' premature triplets, Aaron,
Finn and Ryan. As you will probably remember this was
at the height of the snow and ice which almost brought
the country to a standstill. Our boys were born by

emergency C-section in Wexford General Hospital after a frantic ninety-minute dash by 4x4 ambulances through eight inches of snow.

The 'Snow Babies', as called by the press, featured in all the newspapers and even made an appearance on *The Late Late Show*. At home, the real hard work takes precedence over everything: 18 bottles, 30 nappies, a packet of baby wipes and 2 or 3 hours of sleep a day, not to mention the washing machine, dishwasher and heating on 24/7. As the boys are my first children I got a baptism of fire on a massive scale, but I wouldn't change it for the world.

John, Dad of 3 & Stepdad of 1, Wexford

When you bring your babies home, be sure to call on family and friends for support, and try and take as much time off in the early days to get into some sort of routine. With twins you will both need to rest and recharge. Try and find a system that works especially with the feeds – which doesn't always mean you both have to be up together feeding the twins at the same time.

Damien, Dad of 2, Dublin

I remember being told by the obstetrician that we were not to expect to have a full-term pregnancy as this seldom occurs with twins. Being the type of guy who would normally leave everything to the last minute, I made sure that once we passed the 34-week mark the nursery was sorted, the big baby purchases were out of the away and my boss was being regularly reminded that from here on in I might have to dash off.

Mike, Dad of 2, Waterford

The Name's 'Bond'
Bonding with your unborn baby

Naturally speaking, when it comes to pregnancy and bonding, mums-to-be have an unfair advantage over expectant dads. Dads-to-be for the most part can often feel ignored throughout the pregnancy and important events such as the scan can make the situation feel more real. This innate 'feeling of realism' gives expectant fathers a sense of connection with their unborn baby, and bonding with your baby – especially in the early stages of the pregnancy – is another way to reinforce and maintain this important connection.

5 simple tips for bonding with your unborn baby

1. **The belly-phone**: Various studies have shown that unborn babies are fully aware of their surroundings and are capable of hearing voices from 21 weeks onwards.

   Simply talking, singing or reading aloud a newspaper article will familiarise your baby with your voice, and it's this same voice that your baby will be able to distinguish and take comfort from following the birth.

   Expectant fathers tend to emit low frequencies that travel well through water, ie amniotic fluid, so a deeper voice should be recognisable by your baby, providing you are in close proximity to your partner's pregnant stomach.

2. **Mozart not Metallica**: Exposing your unborn baby to music builds more than just a strong bond; it can also help stimulate your baby's developing brain. Studies have shown that babies prefer classical music as it is said to mimic the mum-to-be's heart rate.

3. **Hands on**: Ask your partner to let you know when your baby is being active so you can feel for any kicks and punches. Also by just resting your hand on her belly, or gently stroking it, baby can feel more at ease and less of a disturbance on a sleep-deprived mum-to-be.

4. **Show her the love**: Scientists have discovered that unborn babies respond to their mother's mood while she is watching a movie – and become quiet and still if the film is sad. The findings, reported in *New Scientist* magazine, add to the evidence that a pregnant mother's mood and stress levels can affect her unborn child. As an expectant father you have a role to play in ensuring that your partner stays relaxed during the pregnancy, though having to contend with raging hormones can be quite difficult at times. Showing love and support to your partner will ultimately filter through to your unborn baby. Practise 'not in front of children' in pregnancy by avoiding any unnecessary confrontation and do your best to attend antenatal scans and classes.

5. **The mail-womb**: Start writing a blog or set up an e-mail address for your unborn child and send them messages to tell them how excited you are, and that you look forward to holding them for the first time.

BUMPEDIA: **FETAL DOPPLER**

A fetal doppler or baby heart monitor is a handheld ultrasonic device that is used to listen to the heartbeat of an unborn child in the womb. Fetal dopplers are used to reassure expectant parents that all is well with their baby. They are effective from ten or twelve weeks into pregnancy, and are easy to use and pose no risk to your baby.

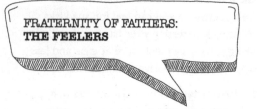

FRATERNITY OF FATHERS:
THE FEELERS

We were both coming home from work on a packed bus when my girlfriend screamed out, 'He just kicked me!' I looked angrily at the man standing up in front of us who said, 'It wasn't me, pal.' To which my girlfriend laughed, 'Not him, you twit, the baby!' It was a bit embarrassing, to say the least, but I'll always remember my son's first kick and the same man who said, 'Can I have a feel?'

Tom, Dad of 1, Dublin

I can remember sitting with my hand on my wife's belly waiting for something to happen and then I'd start to get tired and I'd take it off, only for the baby to kick just at that moment. It was as if he was playing a game with me. I could actually see him doing it. I'd even say, 'I'm taking my hand away', and he'd still wait until it was off to do it again – he must have had eyes looking out of the belly button! To this day he is still that cheeky little boy who constantly keeps his daddy on his toes.

Patrick, Dad of 2, Offaly

Small Change
The price of parenthood

Surely something so small couldn't cost so much. Are you familiar with the proverb 'an extra mouth to feed'?

There are many certainties when it comes to parenting, the main one being a new baby will require regular attention and feeding, and whilst this can be exhausting on new parents, there is still one basic certainty that can elude many novice or expectant parents – the actual cost involved in having a baby.

Budgeting for your baby's arrival should be treated with the same level of importance as choosing the actual baby name. Similarly, it will involve lists containing essential and non-essential items, negotiation, flexibility and personal sacrifices on both sides – especially as up to this point you may have both been financially independent of each other.

Over the kitchen table

Organising a regular pow-wow over a glass of Chablis (or non-alcoholic beverage for your pregnant lady) will give you an opportunity to look at your household income and your expenditure. If you find that your expenditure exceeds your income, you may need to cut back on costs. Discussing your family finances will condition you to keep up this habit after your baby is born, enabling you to manage your finances and allowing you to be more knowledgeable on what it is you can and cannot afford.

Other factors that will need consideration include medical expenses, eg obstetrician fees (private patients), loss of earnings due to maternity leave, childcare costs or whether one parent decides to stay at home and the relevant benefit entitlements.

Savvy saver

Prior to the birth, try to put aside what you can afford in a high-interest savings account; this way any financial surprises that may occur following the birth are already catered for.

 For additional information log on to:
www.ccpc.ie to compare Irish deposit accounts.

The cost of clutter

A shoebox is not a fitting stable for a new baby. All of a sudden you may find that there is no room at your inn to accommodate a new tenant, never mind all its belongings. It is clear that something has got to give, or go. Having a baby presents an ideal opportunity to de-clutter your home; in fact there is money to be made in the process. Take an amble about your abode and before long you will have a list of items from exercise bikes to golf equipment that money can be made from.

Brand new

We can all agree that we want the very best for our children, but there is one major trap that new expectant parents fall into: it is adopting the concept of 'we must get everything, it must be new, and it should be branded'. If expectant couples travel down this weary path (with their Victoria Beckham travel system in tow!) it will end up hurting their finances more than the actual childbirth itself (and that's without pain relief!).

Seconds away

In the very likely event that you hear the following beautiful words being spoken, 'I have a load of baby clothes that I no longer want' or 'I have a baby-changing station taking up space in our attic' – everyone does, believe me! – seize the day with a big fat 'Yes, please'. And while we're on the subject of freebies, throw about the word 'baby shower' during the pregnancy and see what happens!

Can't buy me love

Babies are born every day into all walks of life. Yes, at times it can be difficult – emotionally and financially – but you do get on with it; you make the necessary sacrifices in your own life to give your child the best start in their life. Having a baby or being a father will change the way you view things. Priorities may need evaluating, but for the most part, aside from the bare necessities, what a baby or child needs most and which costs nothing, is the priceless love and attention of his parents.

A Wolf in Sheep's Clothing
Choosing the right family car

Motors are very much mathematical objects. Let me explain. Take a new baby; add the multi-functional travel system, an over-bulging changing bag, a car seat, the weekly shopping and two sleep-deprived parents. Now step back and take a look at your 2-door Audi TT or Mazda MX5 – it's not going to happen, even if you decide to forgo the travel system and wear a sling until they're teenagers!

When it comes to buying a family car, sacrifices have to be made. At some point it will become necessary to trade-in the coupe and turn your sights towards a 'practical' alternative mode of carriage for the family.

Buying your first family car does not necessarily mean your driveway will suddenly be ashamed to hold an unassuming people-carrier. The majority of motoring brands today have designed, and disguised for that matter, a variety of family models to cater for all tastes and fashions irrespective of whether Daddy or Mammy is in the driver's seat. However, there are more important factors to consider than how you look behind the wheel when deciding on a new family car. These include:

Safety first

Safety is of paramount importance to all parents when it comes to choosing a new family car. Whether you are buying a new or used car, you can compare the crash safety ratings of different makes and models on the European New Car Assessment Programme website www.euroncap.com.

Space Invaders

There is a great deal of baggage involved with babies and children; this is why space, with an emphasis on the boot, and a plentiful supply of compartments and cubby holes is essential.

Look at the 'Estate' of you!

Something for all the family – 5-seaters, 7-seaters, SUV, MPV, Estate, Crossovers. Look at the big picture: holidays, comfort, ease of access and ferrying friends. Pay special attention to bench-type seats which are common in some SUV 7-seat models as they may only be suitable for younger children.

Reliability

The issue of reliability is fundamental. Aside from the test drive, owner reviews make it easier for you to arrive at your final decision. JD Power surveys car owners in many countries to see which brands and models have the best quality and reliability records.

 For additional information log on to:
www.jdpower.com

Fill her up

With unstable petrol and diesel prices, fuel awareness is high on everyone's list. However, pulling a heavy cart may require a few horses.

'The power and glory of a high-horsepower engine might sound like fun, but family transporting is generally a period of many short journeys, so choose an engine that is a good lugger. That's where modern diesels score well, with good torque and easy on the wallet,' says Brian Byrne, Editor of *Irish Car + Travel* Magazine.

Take your seats

View any potential candidates with more than one child in mind. Consider that three individual rear seats are mandatory to your selection criteria especially if you are to factor in car and booster seats adjacent to each other. Choose a car that has a full lap and diagonal belt in that seat, as it protects better than a simple lap belt.

Every year children are killed or seriously injured on our roads – often because they are not properly restrained when travelling. According to the AA Motoring Trust, ensuring a child is properly restrained in a child car seat can reduce injuries by a factor of 90–95 per cent for rear-facing seats and 60 per cent for forward-facing seats.

If you're shopping for a new car, bring the car seat (and travel system) with you to test how easy it is to use and be sure to avail of the fitting service provided by your authorised car-seat retailer.

iDad: **WHAT EXACTLY IS ISOFIX?**

Isofix is an international car-seat safety system which was fitted as standard in most new cars since 2006, operating through points on the back of the child car seat that plug into ISOFIX fittings in the car which create a solid link between your child's car seat and your own car, eliminating the need to use the adult seatbelts to restrain the car seat.

The best way to find out if your car has ISOFIX fittings is to contact your vehicle manufacturer or the dealership or simply your car's manual which should highlight the ISOFIX fitting points.

Older cars that don't have ISOFIX installed can use a base and seatbelt to hold a car seat in place; however, your car seatbelt should hold it firmly in place with little movement, and the buckle should never rest on the car-seat frame.

Pass the wipes!

Vomit, leaky nappies (yikes) and ice cream are just some of the ingredients of the everyday family car life, so unless you plan to shrink-wrap the upholstery, being precious about the interior should be the last thing on your mind.

'It might sound a little extravagant, but consider the leather option, if there is one, when buying. Leather is easily cleaned, hard wearing, and does not hold smells. Otherwise, look at industrial-strength, cleanable car-seat covers like taxi drivers often use,' adds Brian Byrne, Editor of *Irish Car + Travel* Magazine.

Finally, the best place to see the biggest selection of different models in operation is in the car park of your local supermarket, crèche or school. Ask your fellow family motorist for their opinion.

Buckle up!
Choosing the car seat

When it comes to travelling by road you should never cut corners with regard to your family's safety. Choosing a car seat is the task that befalls many expectant dads, with mum-to-be only too happy to assign the mission.

If you find yourself in a field of fathers, tugging at straps, dumbstruck by reclining swivel chairs, or bewildered by the notion of ISOFIX, there is a certain protocol to follow when choosing the appropriate car seat:

- Don't buy a second-hand car seat; you cannot be sure how it has been used or if it still complies with safety standards.

- Purchase a car seat from a retailer which provides a fitting service.

- Whatever type you buy, don't wait to fit it for the first time just before you go and collect your newest addition from the hospital. Have a test run a week or so before the birth.

- With the majority of Irish maternity hospitals insisting that new parents take their baby home in a correctly fitted car seat, buying a car seat before your baby arrives can be difficult especially when you are not certain of baby's weight and size. It is best advised therefore to always ask the experts in the shop for their advice.

- Ask other parents to recommend a brand, and remember you get what you pay for – so consider taking from another part of the budget to buy that more expensive model.

- Ensure that your chosen car seat is equipped with a head hugger or head-cushion insert which prevents any head-floppiness.

- Consider every car that your child will travel in before choosing your child seat. ISOFIX seats can also be used with the adult belt if you'll travel in another car without fixings.

- Many parents use the car seat to carry their baby to places they do not wish to take a pram. Check the carry handle is comfortable and that the seat is not too awkward to take out and about – and remember, the seat is likely to be lighter without a baby inside of it!

- Don't modify the seat in any way as this could have very serious consequences in an accident.

Know the law: child car seats

Making sure you use a child car restraint may be the most important thing you do for your child. In Ireland, as many as 4 out of 5 child car seats are incorrectly fitted, which can lead to serious injury or even death in a collision. EU child safety protection laws make it compulsory for all children to travel in the correct child seat, booster seat or booster cushion. The law on child car seats states:

- Where safety belts have been fitted they must be worn.

- Children under 3 years of age must not travel in a car or goods vehicle (other than a taxi) unless restrained in the correct child seat.

- Children aged 3 years or over who are under 150cms in height and weighing less than 36kg (ie generally children up to 11/12 years old) must use the correct child seat, booster seat or booster cushion when travelling in cars or goods vehicles.
- Children over 3 years of age must travel in a rear seat in vehicles not fitted with safety belts.
- Rearward-facing child car seats must NEVER be used in the front passenger seat of cars with an active airbag.
- Child car seats must be in accordance with EU or United Nations-Economic Commission for Europe (UN-ECE) standards.
- Drivers have a legal responsibility to ensure passengers aged less than 17 use the correct seat, booster seat, booster cushion or seatbelt.

Source:
Road Safety Authority (RSA): www.rsa.ie

iDad: **PRINCESS ON BOARD**

A badge proclaiming your fertility can irritate other motorists. Yet, whether you consider them tacky or arrogant, 'Baby on Board' signs are a warning symbol for emergency services that a child may be an additional passenger within a vehicle.

Group deals

When your baby reaches at least 20 lbs (9kg) in weight (between 9 to 12 months), they may start to outgrow their first rearward facing car seat, group 0+, and may need a forward-facing seat, known as a Group 1 car seat.

However, it is best to keep your baby in a rearward facing seat for as long as possible, bearing in mind that your baby's head should **never** reach over the top of the seat, especially if it is a group 0+ seat, and her weight does not exceed 29lbs (13kg).

iDad: **DON'T BE AN AIRHEAD**

Never put a baby in a rearward facing seat in the front of the car without turning off the passenger airbag.

Forward-facing seats will last your baby until they reach 40lbs (18kg), at around four years. These Group 1 seats are much larger and heavier than your baby's first car seat and are designed to be left in the car. Some have a five-point baby harness and use the car's seatbelt to hold the seat firmly in place. Other newer and lighter Group 2 models can be used with the car's own seatbelt reaching across your child, like an adult's seatbelt, and locking it into place.

Size matters

The correct car seat is dependent on your child's height and weight, **not their age.**

Rearward-facing baby seat

- **Weight range**: for babies up to 13kgs (29lbs)
- **General age range**: from birth to 12–15 months
- **Seat details**: provide protection for baby's head, neck and spine

Forward-facing child seat

- **Weight range**: for kids 9–18kgs (20–40lbs)
- **General age range**: 9 months–4 years

Booster seat

- **Weight range**: 15–25kgs (33–5 lbs)
- **General age range**: 4–6 years

Booster cushion

- **Weight range**: 22–36kgs (48–79lbs)
- **General age range**: 6–12 years
- **Seat details**: You must use the seatbelt in conjunction with the booster cushion

iDad: **What is i-SIZE?**

The key benefits of i-Size-standard seats are that they can be fitted to most ISOFIX systems and they provide increased support for the child's head and neck. They also provide better side-impact protection in the event of collisions.

 Source: Road Safety Authority (RSA)
www.rsa.ie

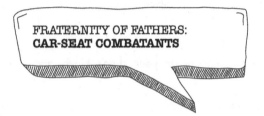

FRATERNITY OF FATHERS:
CAR-SEAT COMBATANTS

At times our little wriggler can silently slip out of his straps, unbeknownst to us up front. We regularly had to stop every mile or so to pull in and re-adjust him. It got to the stage that we had to fit a bigger rear-view mirror just to catch him in the act. We also found that bringing along some toys to distract him from doing a Houdini or saying the car would not go until his arms were back in the straps worked well too.

Mark, Dad of 1, Roscommon

I noticed when we were on holidays that the belt had become twisted and no matter how much I pulled at it, it would not straighten out. Thankfully, at the time of buying the seat, my wife insisted that we put the instructions in the glove compartment which pointed at something not at all connected to the seatbelt as being the problem.

Paul, Dad of 2, Dublin

I considered car-seat covers to be for family pets, but they are very useful in avoiding any spillages by the young folks getting through to your upholstery or tarnishing the leather.

Ivor, Dad of 2, Clare

My routine for checking the air in my tyres also includes checking that the car-seat fitting has not been compromised in any way.

John, Dad of 3, Dublin

Anytime we travel abroad we always check with the car rental company that the correct (& legal!) car seat is being supplied and is already fitted in the car before collection. Similarly, if we are being picked up at the airport by taxi, we usually book ahead or ask our rep to ensure our mode of transfer is fitted with a car seat. In addition, when it comes to car rentals or taxi hire, pay special attention that each has sufficient space to cater for your luggage and pram.

David, Dad of 3, Cork

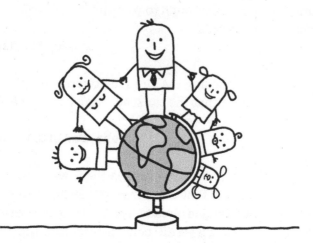

'I cannot think of any need in childhood as strong as the need for a father's protection.'

Sigmund Freud

3 The Third Trimester

The final stretch

Trimester 3: Weeks 28–Birth

The end is in sight as you head into the third trimester. Things are moving fast now; everybody has their own tasks to attend to. For your baby it is a time when she becomes 'engaged' – I know, they start so young! Mum doesn't know whether she's coming or going. One minute she's wobbling uncomfortably towards an inviting armchair, the next she is in the shed looking for your painting overalls. No doubt your own pockets are laden down with lists; there's not much space left on the calendar to cross off now. I can almost hear you sing 'here we go, here we go, here we go' as you dart out your door to another baby emporium in search of the next dadget on your list ...

Womb with a view

In the final stages of the trimester your baby will be less active as she settles into the birthing position – 'head down' in your partner's abdomen, nearer to the pelvis. Your baby is developing rapidly in the third trimester and the good news is that if she is delivered before full term is reached, she will more than likely survive. The chequered flag is waved at the end of the third trimester with labour and the birth of the baby.

Baby talk

'Look at me – I can blink, close my eyes, turn my head, grasp firmly, and respond a lot more to sound, light, and touch – so put your hand back on her belly and raise the volume there on your new Spotify Baby playlist. I know, I'm being a nuisance in here, switching positions and kicking about, but since I've piled on the pounds in the last few months there's not much room, but mum should still feel me every day. That fine hair (lanugo) I had before is falling off big style. Hold on a second, what am I doing upside down. Help! I'm stuck. Ah well, just enough time to pop my thumb in my mouth.

'During this trimester I've folded up the cross-trainer and so my weight has trebled, so don't be surprised if I weigh between 6lbs 2oz (2.78kg) and 9lbs 2oz (4.14kg) when you see me in the flesh. I can also tell you that, since space in here is premium, I reckon from tip to toe I measure between 19in (48cm) and 21in (53cm).

'Anyway Pops, I've heard that size doesn't really matter. As long as I'm healthy that's what's important. Look forward to seeing you soon. Take care of Mum for me.'

Mum's the word

The result of baby's recent expansion will no doubt begin to cause serious discomfort for your partner. This is a physically and emotionally challenging time for her and she may find even doing the most simple of tasks difficult, including getting some much-needed rest. You can help her here by monitoring her sleeping position, ensuring that she is resting on her left side. She can achieve this by placing a pillow between her knees or behind her back which prevents her from rolling backwards.

She may also feel uncomfortable about her appearance, so be kind and keep the quips about 'size of houses' to yourself. While we are on the subject of houses, don't be horrified if you come home from work only to find your better half balancing on the top step of the stairs with a paintbrush in hand, attempting to touch up a spot that only a contortionist could reach – this is nesting!

Medical experts recommend that pregnant women should take maternity leave at 36 weeks. In Ireland at least 2 weeks and not more than 16 weeks leave must be taken before the end of the week in which the baby is due.

Symptom sympathy

By the end of the third trimester your partner may be suffering from shortness of breath, swollen ankles, fatigue, constipation, varicose veins, heartburn and haemorrhoids – basically you name it, and she's most likely to have it! And with baby continuously pressing down on her bladder you'd better make arrangements to use the outside loo!

A new experience for her during the final stage of pregnancy will be the dress rehearsal of contractions known as Braxton Hicks which signals that her body is preparing itself for labour. In contrast to 'real' labour contractions, Braxton Hicks contractions are 'usually' painless.

Plan of action

The third trimester does not give you the opportunity to sit around. There's the birth plan to be drafted, which covers all manner of important issues from birthing positions to feeding methods and change-of-mind clauses (eg for pain relief). There's the invaluable antenatal class to attend (you see, I gave you the benefit of the doubt and didn't say 'classes'!); you have your own manternity bag to pack, and a shopping list of baby essentials has to be acquired and assembled (yikes!).

What's most important in the third trimester is that your heavily pregnant partner can count on her go-to-guy more than ever, so pick up the slack, have yourself an energy drink and show her that if she's impressed with how you are supporting her now, just wait until she sees you when the main event kicks off.

BUMPEDIA: **TELL ME MORE ABOUT BRAXTON HICKS?**

A type of labour contraction in 'training', Braxton Hicks are the body's way of preparing for labour. A woman will not normally feel a Braxton Hicks contraction until the third trimester. They differ from actual labour contractions as they will often disappear if a pregnant woman changes activity.

Braxton Hicks are a part of pregnancy and therefore not a real cause for concern. However, if they are accompanied by other symptoms such as bleeding, loss of water or a slowing down in your baby's movements, medical advice should be sought.

'I Love It When a Plan Comes Together ...'
The birth plan

I have to admit that when I first heard about the notion of birth plans I imagined scented candles and whale music – how wrong I was, well kind of ...

Birth plans play a pivotal role in the act of childbirth. There are choices, decisions (and positions!) that your partner will have to consider in coming up with a birth plan that suits 'her' – one that makes childbirth a comfortable, less stressful and more manageable experience.

A **birth partner** who is familiar with the birth plan will be able to convey certain instructions to the midwife that his partner may for some reason (pain being the obvious one!) be unable to do herself.

**The following are the main items contained
in a birth plan:**

Location: home or away

Today the majority of births in Ireland take place in the maternity ward of your local hospital. The obvious benefits of a hospital birth are that should there be any unfortunate complications with the birth, the equipment and the medical staff are to hand.

However, home births provide your partner with the security of familiar surroundings in a more natural environment. If your partner does opt for a home birth, she will more than likely discuss this with her GP first so they can assess her pregnancy to see if it is suitable.

Birthing positions: on all fours

When we think of childbirth we automatically see members of the opposite sex lying on their backs with their knees up to their ears in an unladylike manner. Yet there are various other positions that your partner can consider – some of which are not only more comfortable for the mum-to-be, but also can actually quicken the process of delivery.

Lying on the back can make it more of an effort to lift the upper body when pushing; it also prevents the use of gravity to help with the birth, as opposed to kneeling on all fours, sitting or squatting. Some maternity wards may also provide birthing pools as sitting in warm water can make your partner's contractions less painful.

Pain relief: it's gas ...

'I am not having an epidural; I tell you I am **NOT** having an epidural ..'

Two contractions later ...

'Get me it right **NOW** or we are finished!'

Should your partner decide to 'change her mind' on her chosen method of pain relief in labour, be supportive and be sure to get it for her **QUICKLY!** Aside from an epidural there are other various methods of pain relief, including 'gas and air', transcutaneous electrical nerve stimulation (TENS) and intramuscular injections such as Pethidine. The midwife attending should be informed as early as possible of your partner's intention to want an epidural.

Couples often consider taking a course of massage, eg Shiatsu, which teaches the dad-to-be to assist in their partner's labour.

The birth partner: Play Robin to her Batman

Witnessing the birth of your baby is undoubtedly one of the biggest, if not the biggest, milestones of your entire life. If you are expecting your first, you are entitled to be a little hesitant and nervous about the whole ordeal. Your partner is going to need someone she can rely on to be supportive and reassuring. If you feel reluctant or are unable to attend the birth, your partner may choose an alternative birth partner, eg her sister, mother or doula.

 WHAT THE EXPERT SAYS: **HIRING A DOULA**

A doula is usually a mother herself who supports couples through pregnancy, birth and the early postnatal period. She's a friendly, familiar face at your hospital or home birth. Her goal is to help the mother and her partner have the best experience possible.

Doulas do not perform any clinical tasks. Hospital midwives are employed by the hospital and are bound by hospital policies. Your doula does not replace your midwife but complements the care your partner is receiving. She is employed by you and is 100 per cent focused on you and your partner's emotional and physical comfort right from the beginning of labour.

The cost of hiring a doula varies, depending on the services being offered and considering the on-call nature of the job – up to two weeks before the couples EDD and up to two weeks after. Some health insurance companies will reimburse a partial amount towards the cost of employing a doula.

Around Ireland doulas and dads are welcomed into the labour ward; however, the Dublin maternity units, in particular, 'prefer' only one partner. Therefore, it is important to discuss your support needs in advance of hospital delivery.

Tracy Donegan is Director of Doula Ireland and author of *The Better Birth Book*

Flexibility: a change of plan

Childbirth can be unpredictable; therefore unexpected events should be planned for. Keep options open and should the plan not go 'according to plan', remember what is most important – that your partner and your baby are safe and healthy.

Some expectant mothers may be advised that a Caesarean section will be needed to deliver their baby; however, a Caesarean may also become necessary if there are complications during labour. If this is the case, medical staff will try to comply as much as possible with your birth plan, but at all times the safety of your partner and your baby will take precedence.

Other key issues to consider in the birth plan include:

- Dad to cut umbilical cord.
- Does your partner want to hold your baby first or let baby be cleaned and swaddled?
- How does your partner feel about the possibility of an assisted delivery, eg induction, forceps, ventouse, episiotomy and the third stage of labour, ie delivery of the placenta?

- ⌗ Decision on feeding.

- ⌗ Duration of stay in hospital.

- ⌗ Do you want your baby's heartbeat to be continuously monitored using a hand-held device (Sonic aid) or electronic monitoring using a belt strapped round mum's waist, or not at all unless necessary?

- ⌗ Special needs, eg religion or diet.

- ⌗ Playlist (no Foo Fighters!).

Short and sweet

Keep the birth plan simple so the midwife can easily find information at a glance. Write or type it clearly and don't write more than one page. When you and your partner have prepared the birth plan give one copy to your midwife/obstetrician a few weeks before the due date, and take additional copies into the maternity hospital with you to hand over once labour commences.

The MANternity Bag
The expectant dad's survival kit

You would think that you are going on holidays (for three weeks!) when you first set eyes on the case at the bottom of the stairs. But this is no ordinary piece of luggage, for this is the 'hospital bag'. Shortly after seeing it, the case itself gives birth to a smaller compact baby one.

The bulging one is assigned for the duration of her stay, and in the majority of situations remains in your car, brought in only after baby is born and mother is in her room. The smaller one is her labour-ward bag which holds the necessary items specific to the delivery suite.

Ordinarily I would not advise you to have a rummage through your partner's personables, but this commandment has a loophole – as her 'birthing partner' you have a responsibility to know what has been packed and, most importantly, where she's packed it! I will spare you a detailed list of what each holds as you have probably seen the 'cutesy-wootsy' booties and babygrows already on display draped across your bed.

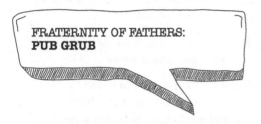

My eldest was born on Easter Sunday when not a shop or pub or hospital canteen was open. We had a very, very long first labour, I say 'we' as I feel that I suffered a little too – I was starving! It made me think that come next time I would be armed with some essentials. Funny though, when the next time did come round, I didn't even get the chance to get the sandwich out of the wrapper!

Kevin, Dad of 3, Dublin

A **'manternity bag'** (patent pending) is an invaluable survival kit for expectant dads containing items that you may wish to consider for your 'own' visit to the labour ward. After all, your partner is a bit too busy to be worrying about making you a sandwich.

The manternity bag can contain:

- **Food & fluids**: Water is essential and high-energy drinks are a good idea. A plain sandwich is a must, but no egg/onion/garlic odours.

- Labour can linger so bring your own **reading materials**.

- **Watch (with stopwatch)**: Not just to count the contractions but also to call the exact moment your newborn enters the world. Check out the various dad-friendly contraction apps on Google Play & iTunes:

oh yes there is an app for everything!'

- ⏹ **Mobile**: Fully charged with credit. Charging bank is essential as you may have many calls to make post delivery.

- ⏹ **Coins:** You may not be able to use your mobile, also useful for parking meters and vending machines.

- ⏹ **Sounds:** This may already be a feature of the birth plan, though soothing, non-ear-bashing playlists only.

- ⏹ **And We're Live**: If you are to venture into reality TV childbirth, don't get carried away with the zoom button and be sure to keep out of the way. It is important, however, that you first check with the attending midwife that the use of recording equipment is within hospital policy.

- ⏹ **A change of clothes/and a basic wash-kit**: You never know when labour may strike and how long it may last.

- ⏹ **The first teddy**: Not fairground size and absent of any tassels and chains!

- ⏹ **Take note:** With all that's going on remember those who helped keep you both at ease during the delivery and hospital stay. A small token of your thanks in the form of a wee box of choccies is guaranteed to get you VIP attention next time round!

Getting Anti about Attending
The antenatal class

 iDad: **WHEN TWO IS BETTER THAN ONE**

Irish expectant fathers have a once-off right to paid time off work to attend the two antenatal classes immediately prior to the birth. This entitlement does not extend to every pregnancy – it's just a once-off right only.

In order to take this time off work, you must notify your employer in writing at least two weeks before classes commence, outlining the dates and times of the classes. Employers can request written evidence of the classes (dates, times, etc).

Antenatal classes prepare you for what is going to occur in the labour ward, helping you to feel less like a tool and a bit more useful than just the guy holding a pregnant hand during labour. You will not be alone; there will be other expectant fathers present.

Most classes take place in the third trimester of pregnancy, so that all mums-to-be in the class are due around the same time. Your partner's GP, obstetrician or midwife will have details of the antenatal classes in your area and in most cases classes take place at your local maternity hospital, but do book early. Private classes in your own home can also be arranged, though these will entail a cost.

Classes take different forms, but for most cases the following are the main areas that are discussed:

- You will learn about the changes to your partner's body and the best way to make life easier for her in the last 12–14 weeks of the pregnancy.

- How to prepare for labour and delivery.

- How to recognise when your partner is going into labour.

- The birth. What you can do to assist your partner, what's going on, and how you can help her relax, including breathing and relaxation techniques.

- Pain relief. Your partner is told what the different types are, when to have them, and the possible side effects.

- Childbirth complications, if labour does not go as planned, eg induction, Caesarean section, instrumental delivery.

- Post childbirth. Parents-to-be receive important advice on caring for a newborn baby, including nappy changing and feeding options.

- Information about all the vaccinations and immunisations your baby receives and the various methods of contraception.

- Antenatal classes also offer a great opportunity to discuss any concerns with the midwife and with other dads-to be.

iDad: **'MANTENATAL' CLASS**

'Mantenatal classes' are courses focused primarily on expectant fathers. Simple massage techniques, how to recognise the signs and stages of labour, your role as the birth partner, and what happens after bringing baby home are some of the topics discussed.

In Australia, mantenatal classes are held in a pub environment where talk of babies is mixed in with the latest sports gossip!

FRATERNITY OF FATHERS:
CLASS CLOWNS

The thought of sitting in a room full of pregnant women talking about babies and childbirth didn't really have much appeal for me, especially as the classes were on Saturday mornings! Anyway, when your partner can get 'emotional' at the switch of a light bulb, digging your heels in is not an option. The classes lasted for just over an hour and we only had to attend two of them, so it was not that bad, really. If it is your first, I would advise it as it does prepare you for what will happen; plus you won't be the only man there.

Gerry, Dad of 1, Dublin

Two things I was not looking forward to – antenatal classes and the birth, but you've got to bite your hand and just do it. It'll be over before you know it. It's one of those things you 'have' to do, like going to the doctor, but once you go, you'll feel better off for it afterwards.

Tony, Dad of 2, Cork

I was glad I did it. My wife's waters broke at home and we had a really fast labour. After arriving at the hospital, I was holding my new baby girl twenty minutes later. It was a close one alright, but had I not attended the antenatal classes I would have been up the walls not knowing what to do.

Patrick, Dad of 1, Wexford

It's not all about breathing exercises; I personally found the information about life at home with your new baby very useful. I also got talking with a few of the other dads on the course which was reassuring to know that we were all in the same boat.

Michael, Dad of 1, Dublin

 iDad: **THE SMALL PRINT**

Check with your health insurance policy for any provisions pertaining to reclaimable maternity benefits/prenatal care/ midwifery services.

In the Thick of It
Attending the birth

If you asked an Irish father in the 70s or even 80s where he was for the birth of his child/ren, he would mostly likely choose one of the following:

- In the pub
- In work
- At home
- In the waiting room

By contrast, today you would be hard pressed to find an Irish expectant father not by his partner's side, or up at her head for that matter. But is there an automatic assumption that expectant Irish fathers 'must' attend the birth? This question is not yours really to answer. It is not us who have the task of giving birth and the impregnated are very much entitled to have whomever they want in their corner, one who will relay information and instructions to the attending midwife/obstetrician and, most importantly, one who can give them the support and encouragement that is so vitally needed in labour, ie the perfect birth partner. Are you that person? Methinks you are.

Naturally, you will be anxious yourself about the whole birth scenario; nobody wishes to see the person they care about suffer in any way. Being prepared for the event will put you more at ease – a little anyway! The antenatal class is the perfect place for this and should certainly be considered, and another is to talk to other dads about their own experiences in the delivery ward.

If you have decided that the birth process is not for you, your partner can request that her mother, sister or a doula attend instead.

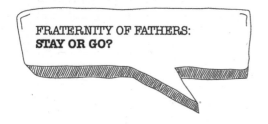

FRATERNITY OF FATHERS:
STAY OR GO?

There was never a question of not attending. I was going to be there to see the birth of my first born no matter what. My boss was very supportive especially as he knew that at any moment I would have to dash off; so in the week my wife was due, we had extra cover put on. When my wife went into labour, it was in the small hours, so it worked out fine. I will say that I am very glad I was present. It is, after all, a monumental occasion in any man's life.

Peter, Dad of 1, Drogheda

How could you not be there? C'mon, it's not as if we had to do much for the nine months, so it's not really a big ask to be there at the birth, as if you didn't want to in the first place!

Gerard, Dad of 2, Clare

I'm a bit squeamish when it comes to blood, and the thought of seeing vast amounts of it didn't really sit well with me. Even after attending the antenatal class I was still very nervous about the whole childbirth side of things. My wife suggested that her sister go in my place which made sense really as I knew she would be a great help in getting her through it all. As it turned out my wife had a quick labour so it only meant that I was not with her for about an hour. If it had been longer, I think I would have begun to regret my decision. If we are fortunate to become pregnant again, I will try and be there next time round.

Martin, Dad of 1, Galway

Times are different now, thankfully, and dads are encouraged to be more involved in the pregnancy, and this is the one place that you can show your support. Having said this, I'm not much of a talker and I don't think I said more than a few words in the delivery ward, just kept out of the way. I did ask the midwife, 'Do most expectant dads attend?' She replied, '99 per cent of the time, the other 1 per cent are not with their partners when they go into labour and get stuck in traffic on the way.'

James, Dad of 2, Dublin

Grounded!
Air restrictions

Air travel is still seen as the safest mode of transportation; however, pregnant women must be fully aware of the obvious pitfalls in travelling at various stages throughout their pregnancy.

It is advised not to fly before 12 weeks or after 28 weeks. The majority of airlines will permit pregnant women up to 28 weeks to fly; after this they will require a letter from their GP confirming their EDD (Expected Delivery Date). The last thing a pilot needs to hear is 'Captain, my wife is going into labour' when he is halfway across the Atlantic – not the type of water birth your partner was hoping for!

There are some airlines which operate scheduled flights that have a more flexible policy in place which can extend up to 36 weeks. Ryanair allows expectant mothers to travel up to 36 weeks with a doctor's letter (**'fit to fly'**) from 28 weeks. For an uncomplicated multiple pregnancy, travel is not permitted beyond the end of the 32nd week of pregnancy.

Be sure to check what type of cover your insurance policy provides with regard to any stipulation on travelling when pregnant, in particular if your partner goes into labour abroad.

If you and your partner do intend to travel by air, the following tips may help her to have a more comfortable journey:

- Flight socks can reduce the risk of DVT (deep vein thrombosis).

- Book an aisle seat for your pregnant partner as she may need to dash to the loo more often than most.

- The aircraft cabin air can be dry; therefore provide plenty of fluids to keep her hydrated (avoid tea & coffee).

- Finally you have an excuse to ring that bell for a few extra pillows: 'Stewardess, my wife is with child, by the way any room up in first class?'

⏺ Do a Riverdance sitting down; it is imperative that she keeps her feet moving to offset any muscle pain or stiffness. It is also recommended for her to do a walkabout every few hours if it is a long haul flight.

What's up, Doc?
Health concerns in the third trimester

Premature labour

When labour starts before 37 weeks of pregnancy, it is termed as **premature labour**. The signs of a premature labour are more or less similar to that of full term labour. Premature babies will need extra help to survive outside the protection of their mother's womb and may stay in the postnatal ward or be placed in a special unit called a Neonatal Intensive Care Unit (NICU), or Special Care Baby Unit.

 For additional information log on to:
www.irishprematurebabies.com

Pre-eclampsia

Also known as toxaemia of pregnancy, **pre-eclampsia** is a serious condition that can arise after 20 weeks of pregnancy. Pre-eclampsia is said to involve a problem with the blood vessels in the placenta and is diagnosed when high blood pressure, fluid retention and protein in the urine are found in an expectant mother. It can occur in 5–10 per cent of pregnancies but is more common during first pregnancies.

Swelling, particularly in the face and hands, often accompanies pre-eclampsia. Other symptoms may include headaches, blurred vision, abdominal pain or nausea and vomiting. Treatment will depend on how close your partner is to her due date and may include bed rest, more fluid intake, additional check-ups and even the possibility of an early delivery.

Placenta praevia

Placenta praevia occurs when the placenta grows in the lowest part of the womb (uterus) and covers all, or part, of the opening to the cervix; in other words, the placenta becomes low lying. This, in turn, makes it prone to bleed which can put both mother and baby at risk. If your partner notices any fresh blood or regular pains, it is important that she contact her GP or obstetrician immediately. An ultrasound will determine the position of the placenta.

In the majority of cases the placenta will correct itself and the pregnancy can proceed as normal. However, if the placenta continues to cover the neck of the womb, your partner may need to have a Caesarean delivery.

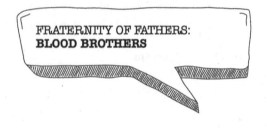

FRATERNITY OF FATHERS:
BLOOD BROTHERS

In April we discovered that my wife Susan was pregnant. We had three boys already; all had been fairly routine pregnancies and, as this was number 4 we were relaxed and looking forward to another arrival in November.

The first hint that this would be a different experience was at Susan's 20-week scan. The sonographer noted that Susan's placenta was low lying and told us that she probably had placenta praevia and queried a condition called Acretta, neither of which I had ever heard of! Susan's obstetrician's approach changed immediately and we were told that this would be a far more managed pregnancy with potential for significant complications.

Boy, was she right! Susan was admitted to hospital at 29 weeks, with a plan to get her to 34 weeks before delivery. The baby however had different plans! On 9 September, Susan had a huge bleed and Sarah was born, 9 weeks' premature, at just 31 weeks' gestation. The baby was born by C-section under general anaesthetic within thirty minutes of the bleed. Both Susan and Sarah were gravely ill afterwards. On Thursday morning, 10 September, Susan was fighting for her life in Intensive Care in one hospital and Sarah fighting for her own tiny life in SCBU in another. Susan had had a massive post-partum haemorrhage and very nearly died. She received thirty-six units of blood and platelets in the ten hours after Sarah's birth. I have no doubt that it was the availability of this blood that allowed fantastic doctors and nurses save her life.

Today, both Susan and Sarah are doing great. It's been a crazy time and we are slowly getting back to normal, whatever normal is with four under eleven!! We feel enormous gratitude to the medical profession and the Irish Blood Transfusion Service and are very much aware of just how lucky we were. I have learnt a lot about blood since then: the average adult has about 10 units; a blood donation has a shelf life of about 35 days, platelets only 5–7 days. Only 3 per cent of the Irish population give blood.

In the four weeks before my daughter's birth, thirty-six A-negative people gave up an hour of their lives to donate blood or platelets; those people gave brilliant medical staff what they needed to keep my wife alive, it's that simple!

I would urge any dads or dads-to-be to think about the day you bring a new baby home from hospital. Blood donors meant that I could bring mum home as well.

Colin, Dad of 4, Kildare

Twigs and Berries
Preparing the nest

Nesting is the term used to describe when pregnant women feverishly rush about cleaning the house in preparation for the new arrival. As the name on the tin suggests, nesting derives from the same primal instinct practised by the majority of the female population of the animal planet.

Though said to be from the result of a combination of biological and emotional factors, one does not have to look too far beyond her yo-yoing hormones for a culprit to blame. Some pregnant women, especially those who have been here before, do not experience this urge and would prefer instead to rest more in the final weeks than to swing from ladders or iron new baby clothes.

Expectant dads often partake in the ritual of nesting – the 'n' in nesting, after all, does stand for 'nursery'. This is your domain; show some enthusiasm and excitement about your impending arrival and get the paint brushes out. If you are unaware of the sex of your baby, creams and yellows are your best colour swatches.

Aside from holding the ladder (ha, ha), now is also the time for you to read up on any instructions that relate to cots, swings, baby seats, breast pumps – trust me you don't want to be doing this on the day you go to collect her from hospital or when she is in the living room giving birth.

Shopping is another side-effect of the nesting mum-to-be, and you will have a duty to accompany her for any remaining baby essentials. Did you really expect her to carry the bags?

BUMPEDIA: **COUVADE SYNDROME**

According to *Scientific American*, **couvade syndrome**, which comes from the French word *'couver'*, meaning 'to hatch', (also called 'sympathetic pregnancy' or 'phantom pregnancy') may affect as many as 80 per cent of expectant fathers.

Couvade syndrome is a condition whereby expectant fathers experience similar symptoms commonly found in pregnancy, eg morning sickness, food cravings and weight gain. Although symptoms are viewed as being 'psychosomatic' (generated by the mind), the physical discomforts associated with the 'condition' are deemed to be very real.

There have been a variety of studies conducted on the topic which show that it may be just a ploy by the expectant father to get some attention or simply an expression of anxiety and fear associated with impending fatherhood. Similarly, some experts believe that couvade syndrome may be occurring more regularly as society's views on fatherhood changes with more men taking a hands-on role in their partner's pregnancy, as well as the birth and the rearing of the child.

Generally the symptoms appear towards the end of the pregnancy, although they have been known to begin as early as the end of the first trimester. Some researchers report that the syndrome is more common in first-time fathers with symptoms disappearing almost immediately after the baby is born.

Kitting out Your Kid
The essentials

Buying baby gear is a lot like choosing items for a wedding list: there are those items that you simply cannot do without, and then there are the items you think you need but only end up using once or not at all. The thing is, you don't pay for the items on your wedding list, but when it comes to buying baby gear, before you can say 'how much?', you're standing over a travel system that costs more than your first car.

Being a dad (or a male), you are bound to be tempted by the latest innovative piece of baby gadgetry, but restrain yourself. Do your homework, ask other parents to list the items they could 'not' do without first, stay within your budget, consider the second-hand option, and never turn down an offer of clothes or equipment – even if they are not suitable for the time being. Most importantly, as with all baby equipment, pay special attention to the safety guidelines as outlined by the manufacturer.

Bedding

Moses baskets are an excellent 'addition' to your baby's sleeping requirements. However, their overall usefulness is dependent on the size of your baby. Parents often choose to avail of a Moses basket for the first month or so until one morning they peek across and see baby's legs swaying over the ends. They are very portable and require a fold-up stand which makes them practical if they need to be moved from room to room. When you consider the length of time they will be used for it is recommended to borrow or acquire one second-hand.

Cots: Times have definitely moved on from the orphan Annie steel-barred enclosures. Today you are bombarded with a wide selection of contemporary **cot** designs with drop-down sides and varying sleeping levels, though the principal goal remains the same – a small but safe jail-like (I know it sounds awful) pen for sleeping beauty.

Cot-beds are exactly what the name suggests, though, be warned, they can in fact work out costing more than your very own king-size, and that's with the silk sheets and Egyptian cotton thread count thrown in! However, when you consider that they can be converted to a bed and last up to five years of age, they do make for an excellent investment. Again, opt for a second-hand one to save a few quid but do ensure that all rails are in working order and that all the bed adjusting hooks are included.

Baby sleeping bags are a great substitute for blankets since they cannot be kicked off, slipped overhead or cause baby's feet to get caught in the bars of the cot. Duvets and pillows, on the other hand, are not recommended for your baby until he is a year old as they can limit your baby's movement and may make him too hot.

Fitted sheets that have elastic going around the entire sheet (not just at the corners) can make life a lot easier for new parents too. In addition, a **mattress protector** can also be placed underneath the cot sheet to prevent any type of leakage finding its way through to the mattress!

 iDad: **BUMPER BEWARE**

Advice from doctors warns that babies can suffocate against, be strangled or trapped by the popular padding or **safety bumper** which wraps around the inside of a cot and ties to slats.

Mattress

Since babies spend 'most' of the time sleeping it is essential that you pay special attention to choosing the correct mattress, quite simply by applying the 4 F's:

Firm: Along with the car seat the mattress is one of the most important pieces of baby equipment you will need to acquire. Speak to an experienced retailer about the different compositions and safety implications of each.

Fit: The cot mattress needs to fit the cot properly. Large gaps can present an unnecessary danger to your child. When pressed tightly against the side of the cot, a mattress should not leave a gap of more than 1.6in (4cm) between itself and the cot sides.

Flame resistant: The ability to retard flames is crucial (as with all equipment types).

First: Though it is recommended to factor in the second-hand option in buying baby equipment or borrowing from family and friends, it is strongly advised that in the case of the mattress, you always buy brand new. In addition, cots and Moses baskets may already come with fitted mattresses so be sure to check the safety standards before buying.

The changing mat and station

A changing mat is an inexpensive wipe-clean item that comes in a variety of baby-distracting colours. Odd as it sounds, a changing station is a raised structure with the mat itself serving as the rooftop with a few handy storage shelves underneath. It's more forgiving on your back than a conventional changing mat, as bending over the bed or getting down on all fours to change junior can cause quite a strain. But be warned: 'Do not leave baby unattended' should be tattooed on your eyeballs whenever you're making use of this piece of equipment.

 iDad: **GET YOURSELF A 'DAD BAG'**
Batman has one, so too does Deadpool. These are superheroes who don't want to be caught out and about with the baby shouldering any floral, brightly coloured changing bag. Well, maybe one of them might! There are a number of macho alternatives when it comes to daddy nappy bags with numerous handy compartments and a travel changing mat. These bags are versatile and discreet in nature so when they are no longer needed for junior they can be transformed into a laptop or weekend bag.

Bath

The ways in which you bathe your baby are more important than the container or tub itself. However, there are a multitude of cradle devices and non-slip bathing mats on the market. Bathing can be a very stressful experience for your baby, so choose the method and mode carefully.

Muslin cloths

If baby gear had an awards ceremony, then the muslin cloth would be the overall winner on the night. It would not only walk away with the award for the 'Most Useful Baby Item' but would pick up the 'Best Dribble Protector' Award (as sponsored by Louis Copeland Suits) and the 'Best Bulk Buy' Award (as sponsored by Musgraves Cash & Carry).

Nappies

The nappy is just the pizza base when it comes down to the changing process. Other ingredients can include wipes, cream, cotton balls, nappy bin/bucket, and scented nappy bags, and when you consider a newborn baby can go through up to 10 nappies a day – you are looking at quite a dent in your household budget, which may have you crying like a ...

The constant battle that exists between 'real' nappies and their disposable counterparts is something of a touchy subject, similar you might say to the sibling rivalry that exists between breast-feeders and bottle-feeders. But whether one fills a landfill and the other wastes water, the final decision will always be dependent on cost, ease of use and comfort.

 iDad: **NAPPY TIMES**

An average child can use up to 5,000 nappies before being toilet trained, and with the popular disposable brands costing 20c each – we're talking about shelling out €1,000 before wee Johnny can pee pee like the big boys.

Clothes

The clue is in the tag. Take a ramble round the rails of any baby store and the first thing that will hit you is that for the first year of a baby's life, the sizes are in months! Listen lads, babies grow – very, very fast. Before you can say '0–3 months' you are reaching for the next shelf of clothes as you wrestle an irate 13-week-old into something that is too big for him now and something that will be too small for him in 4 weeks' time! Why else do they call them babygrows?

Baby clothes are the one thing you can be sure that other parents a) have an EU butter stockpile of, and b) will be over-eager to dispense with. Gifts and donations will largely take care of baby's wardrobe for the first few months. If you decide not to find out the sex of your baby, then neutral colours such as white and yellows are the best option. Don't pay any heed to colours of second-hand items – at 4am, it'll make no difference whether it's pink or blue; after all it's not as if he's going out dancing!

Monitor

When you do see an expectant dad in a baby store you are most likely to find him either examining an upturned travel system or testing the clarity of a baby monitor. With the latter he will carefully scrutinise all the technical information, flipping over boxes to compare features, emanating a similar level of concentration to a new mobile phone purchase.

Baby monitors do offer parents a great deal of peace of mind; equally, they can become the bane of your life as you tether on the edge of your bed, waiting patiently for the next exhale – makes you think how 'irresponsible' our own parents were standing at the bottom of the stairs!

As with mobile phones, the more you are willing to shell out, the more features you can expect to have, including temperature gauge, talkback, mood lighting and video monitoring operated from phone or second monitoring unit.

Prams, Trams and Automobiles
Choosing the right wheels

At last, something for expectant dads to get their teeth into. The buggy, the pram, the stroller, the pushchair, the travel system, the three-wheeler ... Call it whatever you want – if it's got wheels on it, then leave it to us guys.

It is a small (and invaluable) contribution to the pregnancy that gets us off the sideline and makes us feel that we actually have something more to do, outside of foot rubs or sourcing the weird and wonderful cravings from the dark unpleasant corners of the planet.

Pushchairs can blow a whopping big hole right out of your baby budget. They require a great deal of attention when you consider the amount of miles you will be pushing them or the number of years and subsequent children they must cater for. I have seen models sit proudly on display in shop windows for unscrupulous four-figure sums with drooling mums-to-be being pulled away by a sarcastic dad-to-be, chuckling 'sure that should come with aircon for that price'.

The pushchair department of your local baby store serves as a safe haven for expectant dads away from the breast pads and Winnie-the-Pooh paraphernalia, where whistling tape measures mix it up with the rustling sounds of well-researched lists. Expectant dads vie for some one-on-one time with the only sales assistant on duty. Buggies are upturned, tyres are kicked, and folding competitions take place with fellow pramees each confident that they have found 'the secret knack'.

 iDad: **STOP TAKING THE MAC!**

Before you go out of the shop thinking that you have a piece of equipment off an F1 assembly line, let me burst your tyre for you: Owen Finlay **Maclaren** was the inventor of the lightweight baby buggy with a collapsible support assembly and **McLaren** Racing Limited, trading as Vodafone McLaren Mercedes, is a British Formula One team.

Having said that though, Owen Maclaren did design the undercarriage of the Spitfire, so you could say his fleet of buggies could be faster than that of an FI car!

5 common pushchair questions asked by expectant dads:

The Great Outdoors:

'I'm an outdoorsy kind of guy, and I see myself pushing junior up in the hills of the Wicklow Way. Can these wheels take the punishment?'

Three-wheel models are suitable for covering varying terrains such as town and country; many have swivel wheels and are fitted with inflatable tyres.

Club him:

'I like a round of golf and my clubs are never far from my side. If they are not in my hand, they are in the boot. When this thingy is folded up, how much room does it take up?'

Enquire with a member of staff about the possibility of testing out the display model in the boot of your car. It is best advised to do this during a quiet period as opposed to a busy, demanding Saturday afternoon.

Pain in the ... back:

'As you can see, I'm quite tall, whereas my partner over there can hardly be seen over your shelves. Are there different-sized prams?'

An adjustable handle is essential for parents of varying heights and can also reduce any discomfort which may result in back pain. In addition, adjustable handles can be used to switch between front- and rear-facing positions, giving a baby or infant a dual viewing gallery.

The reassurance that they can see a parent when in reverse can send them off to the land of nod; alternatively, any activity happening out in front can serve as a distraction and keep baby awake until the next feed.

What's included?

'It's what they say when you buy a beamer: you buy the engine – the extras are extras. Besides what I see here in front of me, what else is included?'

Though the tag will often itemise what is included in the price, items such as foot-muffs, parasols or rain-covers are additional accessories that can be purchased separately.

Can I have your word on that?

'The better half wants to go again after having this one, so this pram will have to do him too. What sort of guarantee do you offer?'

A pushchair is a big purchase and if you are paying a high price you will expect quality. You will also assume that should more children come along, the pushchair will stand the test of time. The guarantee is therefore very important and that is why many retailers offer more than 1 year.

A pram for every man:

TRAVEL SYSTEMS	STROLLERS	3-WHEELERS	DOUBLES/ TANDEMS
Suitable from birth	Not recommended from birth	Check suitability from birth	Usually suitable from birth
Can be used with an infant carrier	Affordable, practical & lightweight	More manoeuvrable than four-wheelers	Suitable for two passengers
Can be switched between pushchair and pram	Folds down for easy storage	Bulky – make sure you have plenty of boot space	Side by side (double) or 'top gun' (tandem) seating
Ease of movement of baby from car seat into pushchair	Great for public transport & holidays	Good suspension/ suitable for all terrains	Due to the double capacity can be a lot heavier and more cumbersome

A quick word in your ear about ... SAFETY

When buying a pushchair, stroller or buggy, look for a model with a five-point safety harness that has straps that go over your baby's shoulders, round baby's middle and between baby's legs for maximum security. Check also the brakes – can all wheels be locked together or just the back ones?

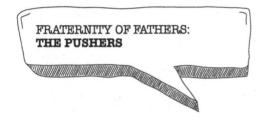

FRATERNITY OF FATHERS:
THE PUSHERS

If you can, try to avoid shopping for baby stuff on the weekend, especially on a Saturday. I can remember the store being packed with moody men who didn't want to be there and foot-tapping pregnant woman eye-balling one another on whose turn it was next. You'd think everyone was due the following day.

Gerry, Dad of 3, Cork

Definitely do your homework, shop around, look at reviews on the web, and ask your mates in work who are dads what pram they bought. It's big money, so take your time and don't be afraid to go back a few times and be sure to ask what's the best deal you can get, especially if you are buying a few other bits 'n bobs from the same store.

Martin, Dad of 1, Dublin

We bought two of the same bases for my wife's and my car. It was handier than switching the one across the whole time. As our daughter got older, her grandparents bought a cheap stroller for their house which meant we didn't always have to take our own when visiting.

Peter, Dad of 1, Galway

Be careful with the size when it's folded. You may be relieved that it actually fits in the boot, but have you considered when you go out where all the other bags are going to go?

David, Dad of 2, Dublin

What's funny is that many of my wife's girlfriends actually try to outdo each other when it comes to having the best pram; they're seen by many yummy mummies as serious status symbols. My wife would joke when we are out shopping: 'that mum over there drives a BMW X5 or Volvo XC90', and sure enough when we are putting the shopping in the boot we see the same mum at her XC90.

Ian, Dad of 2, Leitrim

I've seen it plenty of times and you'll be tempted to do it yourself: when your hands are full you'll start to suspend bags and jackets off the handles. If you do, the buggy will end up doing a wheelie and baby's head may hit the floor. There is nothing worse than turning away for a split second only to hear this God-awful sound and a crowd of onlookers with their hands to their faces – Daddy of the Year, I don't think so …

Conor, Dad of 2, Louth

Strollers are great; I rank them up there for their versatility and usefulness along with pocket raincoats, and in fact there are certain models that are permitted on aircraft as carry-on luggage.

Brian, Dad of 3, Cork

Recommended sites for pre-owned baby equipment:

www.adverts.ie
www.babymarket.ie
www.donedeal.ie
www.ebay.ie
www.jumbletown.ie
www.thestorkexchange.ie

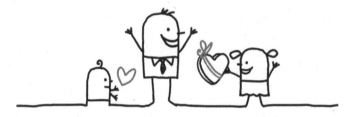

'I felt something impossible for me to explain in words. Then, when they took her away, it hit me. I got scared all over again and began to feel giddy. Then it came to me ... I was a father.'

Nat King Cole

4 Labour

The main event

Congratulations, you have reached the final level. As the due date nears you begin to rub your hands together as if gearing up to deliver the baby yourself.

At this stage, the only communication you have with your partner consists of, 'Will we ring the midwife?' 'How do you know it was just wind?' 'I can't sleep either.'

You begin to eye up the expected date of delivery with a great deal of suspicion. Maybe they got it wrong; hold on a second, was I away on business nine months ago? Now here come the 'what if's' ... What if the car breaks down on the way to the hospital? What if something goes wrong in the delivery room? What if my baby doesn't like me?

All these thoughts and feelings are part and parcel of the pregnancy, especially the weeks up to, or days following the due date – every expectant dad goes through this. The closer you are to seeing your new baby, the bigger the build-up of tension. This chapter will do its utmost to puncture any apprehension you may have towards childbirth.

Show Me the Baby ...
Signs that she is in labour

a. She has a 'show' – not the pantomime sort!

b. There's a puddle on the floor!

c. She is having period-like cramping pains accompanied by backache

All good answers and all correct.

a. You're making a 'show' of me ...

A 'show' is a small leaky discharge made up of blood and mucous that 'shows' itself after the mucous plug sealing her cervix is released. If your partner is having any sort of bleed (even if you suspect it is the 'show'), contact her midwife or maternity hospital.

b. Pass the kitchen roll, honey ...

As you will know by now, your unborn baby develops and grows inside a bag of fluid called the amniotic sac. When the membranes of this sac rupture the fluid will start to leak. It may flow like Niagara Falls or trickle out like a leaky tap, but once her waters have broken, she will continue to leak fluid for the duration of her labour.

A word of warning, amniotic fluid should be clear or have a pinkish hue. If baby has opened his bowels, releasing meconium (baby pooh), then the fluid is most likely to be green/black. If this is the case, contact your midwife/maternity hospital immediately as this may indicate that your baby is in some form of distress.

Speaking of puddles, your partner may feel the urge to use the loo a bit more in the run-up to labour; this pressing down on her bladder is an indicator that your baby has dropped into position.

c. Contraction-ally bound

I have been 'informed' by the mothering masses that contractions first raise their ugly head in the guise of a bad period pain with a gradual cramping across the abdomen often accompanied by backache. Unlike Braxton Hicks, bona fide contractions are those that render your partner powerless to move or speak until they have passed on by (no, they can't be bought on the internet for future arguments!).

Start timing the length of her contractions, taking note of the frequency, and if they remain regular. If you have a level of trust that surpasses any celebrity relationship, then I dare you to get a little closer to the action: Place your hand on her abdomen to feel when it gets hard; when the muscles relax you will feel the hardness ease. Be warned, watch out for her own spare hand; you may find it lodging in the side of your face.

Your partner will more than likely be in labour if the contractions last for more than half a minute and begin to arrive closer together and get stronger. At this stage, call the midwife or maternity hospital to make them aware of the situation.

Was it? Is it?

The majority of women will know themselves when they are in labour. It will be a unique experience for each woman and will differ from birth to birth. On the other hand, first-time mothers (and over-eager dads) have confessed to being a little over-zealous when it came to reacting to activity downstairs – especially occurring around the expected date of delivery. Novice expectant couples will race off to the maternity hospital or ring their midwife (in a home birth situation) only to be told when they arrive and are examined that they are still in early labour and must return home.

This can be quite disheartening on an expectant couple who have left their front door a short while earlier with an 'it's time, here we go' attitude. This enthusiastic approach to childbirth, however, should not be ignored. Should your partner have any concerns about her pregnancy, contact your maternity hospital or midwife immediately – it's what they are there for.

Try to remain positive. Your journey has started; it may take a little more time, but there is no going back now!

If you are told to return home or if contractions are still far apart:

- ☐ Don't just slouch down on the coach in a huff, tapping the remote.
- ☐ Prepare some food for you both.
- ☐ Pop on a girlie flick.
- ☐ Go over the birth plan.
- ☐ Contact family to inform them of the situation.
- ☐ Time her contractions.
- ☐ Encourage and participate in her breathing exercises.
- ☐ Keep her spirits up by showing her some affection.

Get that Kettle Away from Me!
How to deliver a baby ...

The Scenario: your partner is having the baby.

Timeframe: very (very) soon or right now.

People Present: excluding your partner, just you!

Location: at home/in car

I will spare you the sleepless nights (there will be enough of those afterwards) by not highlighting any facts and figures of emergency deliveries that are performed by spouses or partners. I will say that it can happen, and that some day you 'may' find yourself assuming the role of deliverer should your partner or an expectant damsel in distress go into labour.

Remember, childbirth is totally natural. What you need to do is to keep the mum-to-be relaxed; her body and the baby will do the rest.

Instructions on how to deliver a baby (no kettle of boiling water required — unless you're making tea!)

1. First off: don't panic! You may want to, but don't. Your principal task is to keep your partner as calm and as comfortable as possible. Talk to her, try never to leave her side or if you need to, continue to shout out instructions so she is reassured that you are still there.

2. Help remove your partner's lower clothing, put some clean sheets down so baby doesn't touch the floor. Mum will need at least one pillow for under her hips.

3. Remind her to breathe deeply and push when she feels like pushing.

4. Contact emergency services and your midwife/maternity hospital for instructions and to inform them of the situation. Be sure to let them know as much information as possible, eg if you are having twins or if you are aware that your baby may be breeched (coming out feet first).

5. Is there anybody nearby? Ask one of the 'open-mouthed-mobile-phone-recording-spectators' gathered around for assistance. If you are at home, contact the friend/family member closest to you.

6. Try to determine how far apart her contractions are; this will give you an indicator of how near she is to delivering. If her contractions are five minutes apart, it is unlikely that she will give birth within the hour. If they're two minutes or less apart, get ready to deliver the baby.

7. Try to clean yourself as much as possible – do you have hand wipes in the car?

8. Once the baby's head has crowned, try to see if the umbilical cord is around baby's neck. If it is, gently loosen it and slip it over the head. Your wife will need to push when her contractions are strong and rest at other times.

BUMPEDIA: **CROWNING**

Crowning is simply when the widest part of the baby's head (or their crown) begins to come out. As it is seen as a precursor to your baby being born, expectant dads are often asked if they would 'like' to experience the moment. It also lets mum know that she is almost there, especially if her partner can provide commentary on the action as it unfolds. However, your partner may feel more comfortable having you by her side, providing encouragement and support in the final stages of the delivery.

9. Support baby's head as it comes out, moving it downwards as she pushes; the shoulders will be next, and mum will continue to push. Once both shoulders are clear, baby should slip right out. If she is having difficulty doing this, you will have to assist to help the shoulders come out. Do not pull on the baby, but guide the shoulders out.

10. When the head has emerged, check to see if baby is breathing correctly. Clear away any mucus around his mouth or nose.

11. After your baby has popped out, and I do mean popped out (have your catcher's mitt at the ready!), lay your baby face down so fluids can drain from the mouth. Wipe away any amniotic fluid or blood from his skin – this will also stimulate him into taking his first breaths.

12. Wrap him in a blanket or jacket to keep him warm. Make sure to cover him from head to toe, but leave the face open so baby can breathe.

13. Do not cut the umbilical cord. If the cord is long enough, have mum lay with baby on her chest.

14. Don't pull out the placenta. If it comes out on its own, wrap it up so it can be examined later. The placenta will still be attached to your baby by the umbilical cord.

15. Off to the hospital. There may still be some important tests to be conducted to ensure baby and mum are fine.

iDad: **THERE WILL BE BLOOD ...**

C'mon, surely you're not that naive. If you are at all squeamish, then you have no business being down below in the first place – stay up on deck.

Speaking of bodily fluids, it may happen that your nearest and dearest may have a bowel movement (a pooh!) during labour. This is understandable when you consider that she is using her lower muscles to push. If this happens and your partner becomes aware of it, ignore it; instead bring her focus back to concentrating on her breathing. Midwives are exceptional in this situation and are incredibly sympathetic and diligent when it comes to removing any indiscretion.

What's up, Doc?
The three stages of labour

Labour is the road travelled on in order to reach the final destination. Now granted, the road can be short or long, hard on the feet or like a cushion of pillows (with the addition of pain relief that is), and can branch off into different directions, especially at the beginning of the journey.

It is also true to say, as so many of us men do, that 'my wife is going into labour' – for labour consists of various stages that pregnant women must go through before cradling their new baby for the very first time.

The first stage consists of the early, active and transitional phases. The second stage of labour is when the pushing starts and your partner gives birth, and the third stage is when the placenta or afterbirth is delivered.

However, every woman's labour is unique; in some cases their labour can last for hours, and in others, can last as far as the receptionist's desk or the back seat of the car!

As labour is very much a physical process, your partner will experience various emotions as she moves through each stage.

She may not be up for full-blown conversation and may begin to communicate less and less as her labour progresses. It is important that you understand and support her, and recognising each stage will help you achieve this.

BUMPEDIA: **THE STAGES OF LABOUR**

The First Stage:

This stage is usually the longest and refers to when your partner's cervix (neck of the womb) begins to dilate (widen). The stage itself is divided into three phases:

Latent Phase:

- The early period of labour when your partner begins to dilate.

- Her contractions are usually mild, can I say tolerable?

- At the end of the latent phase her cervix dilates to approximately 3cm to 4cm. It is at this point you should contact your maternity hospital to make them aware that you are on your way.

Active Phase

- This is the time when her labour contractions are much stronger and more regular.

- Contractions occur around three or four minutes apart and last up to a minute or so.

- An internal examination may be conducted to determine baby's position.

- The cervix may dilate to about 6cm or 7cm.

Transition Phase

⏍ Her contractions become more intense and painful.

⏍ It may feel that the period between contractions has decreased or that there is no break at all.

⏍ Your partner may feel the need to go to the toilet or push even though complete dilation may not have taken place.

⏍ The cervix may take around an hour or so to dilate to 10cm.

⏍ The transition phase averages between 1 to 3 hours and can be shorter for mums who have given birth before.

The Second Stage:

⏍ The active part of labour when your baby will be delivered.

⏍ Her waters may break naturally or are ruptured by an attending midwife or obstetrician.

⏍ The cervix is fully dilated to 10cm.

⏍ Contractions are extremely strong and come every 2–3 minutes. She may feel that the second contraction starts before the end of the first one.

⏍ This stage can last for as little as 10 minutes for someone who has previously had a vaginal birth to two to three hours for a first-time mum.

⏍ If your partner has had an epidural and cannot feel to push, you can help by placing a hand at the top of her tummy to feel when the contractions start and finish for her, so she can push normally.

⏍ An episiotomy may be performed to assist with the birth (more on that later).

⏍ Assistance may be required for the delivery in the form of forceps or ventouse (vacuum).

⏍ This is your opportunity to encourage and support her as she will naturally feel exhausted – help her to sit up, give her a drink through a straw, and/or sponge her brow.

- You are also best placed to tell her what's going on down below.

- Once the head has emerged, the delivery staff will turn the body to deliver the shoulders next. The rest of the baby will then slip out.

The Third Stage:

- This is where the placenta (baby's nourishment for the last nine months) is delivered and checked to ensure it is complete.

- She may be administered an injection which helps the placenta come out. This quickens up the third stage and will require little, if any, pushing.

- Understandably your partner may not even notice that this stage has occurred, being very much distracted with your new baby. She will also be a tad exhausted!

- Episiotomy or tear will be repaired.

Tongs of Praise
Assisted deliveries

There are situations in childbirth when intervention, or an assisted delivery, becomes necessary. This includes:

- If baby is in any form of distress (sounds like his dad alright!).

- Baby is keeping his mum in labour and refuses to travel the last leg down the birth canal (this stubbornness he gets from his mother's side!).

- If baby is being awkward and has put himself in a difficult position (being awkward – easy, like his mother-in-law!).

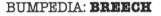

BUMPEDIA: BREECH

Most babies lie in a head-down position in the womb and will emerge head first; however, some babies lie in the 'breech' position – referred to as bottom or feet first.

To 'nudge' the baby along, obstetricians or midwives often use two oversized household utensils: a pair of Gulliver's salad tongs, timidly known as a 'forceps'; and a 'Dyson' with a miniature helmet on the end called a ventouse (your linguistic skills are correct, it is indeed French for 'cupping glass'). Both apparatuses serve the same function – that is, to 'ease' the baby down the birth canal.

In order to insert said item into the birth canal, your partner may need an episiotomy. The following explanation of an episiotomy may emit a large degree of male flinching, notwithstanding oceans of sympathy for your pregnant partner:

BUMPEDIA: EPISIOTOMY

The scientific term describes an episiotomy as a cut to the area of tissue between her vagina and anus. Slicing this area of the female nether region enlarges the vaginal opening, thus enabling the midwife/obstetrician to create more room for baby to pass on through. She will be given pain relief in the form of a local anaesthetic injection inside of her vagina. As forceps can cause more tearing, it is more likely that the midwife/obstetrician will try a ventouse first.

I could just about handle venturing down to the action to see our baby being delivered, but I will never make the mistake again in walking about after the birth in a daze only to turn and witness the obstetrician in all his glory suturing my wife after an episiotomy – gunshot wound is an understatement!

Leo, Dublin, Dad of 1

When your baby is finally delivered, don't be taken aback should she have a misshapen or cone-like dome – this can happen with an assisted delivery especially in the case of a ventouse extraction. The shape of the head will usually return to normal within weeks or months of birth.

Your partner will undoubtedly be quite sore from internal bruising caused by a forceps delivery; she may also require stitches following an episiotomy or tear which should heal within a few weeks. Post pregnancy 'bump-bump' may have to be put on the back burner for quite a while. If, however, you are feeling hard done by, then I advise that you skip back and read the definition of an episiotomy!

My wife had been pushing for nearly an hour and was extremely exhausted especially as her contractions had started to appear the previous day. After seeing my wife in such distress, I suggested to the attending midwife that she may need a little 'extra' help. Our midwife suggested ventouse and thankfully after a short time our baby girl was delivered. Afterwards, my wife said she was amazed (and grateful) that I took charge and appreciated that the decision to have an assisted delivery was in her and our baby daughter's best interest.

Michael, Dad of 1, Waterford

Exploring Other Avenues
Caesarean section

According to the Department of Health, Ireland continues to have higher Caesarean section rates than the EU average, with a rate of 27 per 100 live births.

Vaginal deliveries are still the most common way to give birth in Ireland; however, a Caesarean section (C-section) is often advised and performed in certain situations, particularly if there are complications or any difficulties in labour (emergency section).

A Caesarean may also be planned in advance (elective section) and can take place one to two weeks prior to baby's due date; this ensures the baby is mature before delivery. This also has its own benefits for the expecting Irish father who can organise his paternity leave/holidays with his employer.

If a C-section becomes necessary during labour, your partner may feel disappointed that she is unable to have the normal vaginal delivery that she had planned for. As her birth partner she will look to you for support and reassurance during this intervention. You may also experience anxiety as you had assumed that the birth would go according to plan. No expectant dad wishes to see his partner or baby in any form of distress, and though a C-section is still a major surgical procedure, it is very much an everyday common occurrence in Irish Maternity Hospitals which can last between 20–30 minutes.

Expectant dads can be present if the operation is being carried out under a local and not general anaesthetic (when your partner is put under). You will, however, be 'scrubbed' up in mask and gown. This will certainly make you feel part of the delivery team, and no, you cannot take your new attire home to brag to your mates that it was you that actually delivered the baby!

The anaesthetist will give your partner a 'local' anaesthetic (an epidural or spinal block). Once this takes effect, the obstetrician will begin the procedure which involves making an incision around her bikini line allowing him/her to deliver your baby through the skin after the womb has been opened. After the placenta (afterbirth) is delivered, the obstetrician will close the incision. It is during this stage of delivery that you will be charged with taking care of your baby.

Caesarean patients may require additional days to recover in hospital. Your partner may also have difficulty moving about, especially with regard to sitting or standing up straight. It is imperative that you help out as much as possible at home in the weeks that follow her surgery.

 iDad: **C-SEXTION MYTH**

It is often assumed by men that if their partners have a C-section, it would help quicken up the process of getting 'back in the saddle' when it comes to having sex, especially as her bits are left intact with a C-section. However, this is not the case. Women who have had Caesareans suffer from the same problems as those women who've had vaginal deliveries, including pain in penetration and intercourse.

Help Wanted
Pain relief in labour

Surely that's not the mother of my unborn child spouting profanities more suited to a Roddy Doyle novel than the calming surrounds of a delivery suite.

Our partners have the final say when it comes to what type of pain-relief methods they will adopt during childbirth. In many cases, our heroine will opt for a natural birth right up to the very moment when things become a little more painful and damn right unbearable!

The birth plan itself may feature specific instructions relating to this matter, though a degree of flexibility should always be allowed for, including any last-minute adjustments or additions.

As her partner, you should be aware of the various options available, should her best intentions disappear at the final hurdle. At the same time, you should encourage and support her, should she find herself changing her mind to alleviate any discomfort she is experiencing during labour.

No partner wishes to see their loved one in pain. It can be very difficult for expectant fathers knowing that they are powerless to do anything about it. This is why reassurance plays an integral role in the act of labour. Reassure your partner that the pain is only temporary and will not last; that an increased level of pain means you are getting nearer to seeing your new baby. Supply a 'contraction distraction'. Try to engage her in minor chit-chat, use a damp cloth to wipe her brow, or offer a drink or loose hand for the squeezing, and, where possible, try to maintain eye contact.

The following are pain-relief options that may be available to her:

Push the button: A TENS machine

A TENS (transcutaneous electrical nerve stimulation) machine is a drug-free, non-invasive pain-relief method that is safe to use for both mother and baby.

TENS is believed to work by encouraging the body to produce more of its own natural painkillers, called endorphins, which help block pain impulses from reaching the brain. It is most effective if your partner plans to give birth at home or is in the early stages of labour.

TENS machines deliver small electrical pulses to the body using electrodes placed on the skin. Electrodes are taped on to the back and connected by wires to a small battery-powered device. Soothing pulses are sent by means of the electrode pads through the skin and along the nerve fibres.

The TENS machine is equipped with dials that can be adjusted to control the frequency and strength of the pulses. There's also a boost button for when a 'difficult' contraction occurs. If you intend to be present at the birth ensure that you are familiar with the instructions of the TENS machine as it will be down to you to attach the pads to your partner in the early stages. Be sure to have one or two rehearsals in the final few weeks of the pregnancy as within the comfort of your home and with the notable absence of contractions the scenario can be a tad different to the main event in the labour ward.

There are no harmful side effects; however, the jury is out on the overall effectiveness of this device with some expectant mothers claiming it was a life saver and others tossing it to one side. Either way, it should be viewed as an instrument for reducing pain and not eliminating it altogether. A TENS machine may be used in tandem with other forms of pain relief such as gas and air.

TENS machines are available to rent or buy from all leading pharmacies nationwide.

A pain in the ass! Pethidine

Pethidine is widely used for pain relief during the first stage of labour. A drug which has a similar effect to morphine, pethidine is administered through an injection in the buttocks or thigh. Acting on the central nervous system, pethidine hinders the pain signals that are sent to the brain, helping your partner relax more, though it can also make her feel nauseous and a 'little out of it'.

The main disadvantages associated with pethidine is that it can cross the placenta (from mother to baby) affecting baby's breathing. Establishing a feeding routine may also be difficult as pethidine can pass into the mother's breast milk as well. If this does occur, your baby may be given an antidote to reverse the effects. Pethidine is best avoided when the birth is close.

I'm entonoxicated! Gas and air

Entonox, or gas and air, is a colourless and odourless gas made up of a mixture of oxygen and nitrous oxide gas, or laughing gas as it is commonly referred to. Available in maternity hospitals and gas bottle form for homebirths, it is most often used in the first stage of labour and is easily combined with other pain-relief options.

Slow deep breaths are inhaled through a mouthpiece, or a face mask, at the first sign of a contraction, numbing any pain, and placing your partner in a more relaxed state. There are no harmful side effects to her or the baby, but it can make your partner feel lightheaded and nauseous.

Some female users swear by it, others swear against it! As your partner is in full control of administering entonox, should you be offered a quick fix when the midwife's back is turned, I would advise that you refrain. Remember, you may have the responsibility of cutting the cord later on, and it's best to be coherent to ensure that it's the cord that you are cutting!

There is a god! Epidural

Contractions are strange things; they should be bottled and used as an instrument of torture in finding out your enemies' top secrets. However, to an unsuspecting first-time mother, their first introduction to a contraction often emits a different reaction: 'Was that a contraction? Not bad at all. I can handle that, so much fuss about nothing really.' Then your eye catches that of the midwife and you can tell that that 'mild-mini-contraction' was only the slow ride up out of the rollercoaster tunnel with plenty of wild dips ahead, each getting bigger and more frequent as she rockets on.

To explain or demonstrate the pain-relief capacity of an epidural, I must make reference to that great singer songwriter of a bygone age, Chesney Hawkes (writer's age indicator!), as this is without any shadow of a doubt the 'one and only' method of pain relief that dads would opt for if they were to have the babies. That's not to say, if we could also have a little gas and air, we'd be laughing!

Epidurals reduce pain more effectively than other pain-relief drugs in labour. It's a type of local anaesthetic mixed with a narcotic that is injected by an anaesthetist between the bones of the spine. The pain relief can then be infused continuously or topped up as required. The epidural numbs the nerves and the ensuing pain of contractions, resulting in a pain-free delivery.

The initial dose takes about 20 minutes to administer and numbness usually results about 20 minutes later. While pain relief can be remarkable, it is not without its drawbacks:

- Epidurals can slow down labour if they're given too soon.

- Being numb from the waist down can make it harder for your partner to feel contractions and push at that integral moment of childbirth.

- Unless she is given a 'walking' or mobile epidural, your partner will be required to stay in bed for the entire labour.

- Epidurals can also cause her blood pressure to drop,

which in turn may slow baby's heartbeat. To prevent this, she'll be given intravenous fluids and will require frequent blood-pressure monitoring and continuous foetal monitoring.

⌀ The need to use a urinary catheter and the transient post labour immobility is another factor to be considered.

⌀ Back pain and headache are another potential complication.

⌀ Epidurals may also increase the chances of a forceps or ventouse delivery.

It is important that you inform your midwife upon arrival if your partner is having an epidural or if she has changed her mind from the 'definitely not' to the 'most definitely' as the anaesthetist may be busy elsewhere.

Relationships have been put to the test on how soon this god-like creature arrives. It's one thing pacing the corridor waiting for news of baby's arrival but pacing the corridor on the lookout for the anaesthetist is a completely different story. I can recall my own wife howling, 'Is he here yet? Can you ring him again PLEASE!!!'

Only the brave: natural pain-relief alternatives

While natural pain-relief alternatives won't offer the same level of relief as say an epidural, there are methods your partner can engage in to make her labour easier, including:

Breathing: Put your antenatal class homework into practice and help your partner to focus on her breathing when a contraction occurs. Breathing in through the nose and out through the mouth. Mimicking the technique in unison with your partner may also help her (and you), but don't be surprised if you are told to keep shtum as you may be putting her off her count through a contraction.

Massage: Another hands-on method for expectant dads to get involved in. Your partner will decide whether it is more comforting before, during or after a contraction. Pay attention to particular areas for relaxation, and go easy – you are not kneading bread; this is a pregnant woman we are talking about!

Walk about or a change of positions: Help keep your partner active by walking around with her. If she's lying down, help her to change position frequently to ease backache.

Water: We all can appreciate a nice warm bath so is it little wonder that an increasing number of pregnant women are turning to water for labour and birth? In addition to pain relief, water provides support to the body, increases relaxation thereby reducing anxiety, decreases tearing and encourages dilation.

Birthing pools are currently not available in all Irish hospitals. If you are booked to tour the labour ward, check on the situation regarding birthing pools. Alternatively, if your partner has chosen to have a homebirth, there are plenty of companies who offer pools for hire, or you could opt for an inflatable version you can pump up at home.

Other alternative methods of natural pain relief include: hypnotherapy, birthing balls, reflexology and shiatsu. If your partner intends to use any of these methods, it is important to discuss it with her midwife or doctor and to let the hospital know beforehand.

Finally, research has shown that when a pregnant woman has someone special with her during labour, to comfort, support and reassure her, she gives birth more quickly and easily than if she doesn't. It is important that you avoid adding to her stress by displaying your own anxiety. You are entitled to feel nervous, but this is not the time to let her see it.

WHAT THE EXPERT SAYS:
ACUPRESSURE IN CHILDBIRTH

Shiatsu Acupressure is a tool which enables expectant fathers to actively engage in their partner's labour. Shiatsu involves hands-on application of pressure to different parts of her body. It is safe and supportive and can even quicken the delivery. The use of Shiatsu Acupressure in labour involves basic techniques and specific points which have been observed to have certain effects on the body. With the help of a qualified practitioner, the basic techniques can be learned in a few hours with most couples attending during the last trimester, usually within 4–8 weeks of their delivery date.

With Shiatsu, from the first contraction to the last push, you can be involved and will be able to help support your partner immeasurably.

Brian O' Leary Lic Acu Dip ESS MTCMCI MSSI is a Shiatsu practitioner and acupuncturist who specialises in fertility and pregnancy Acupuncture and Shiatsu.

I Like It in Here ...
Natural methods for bringing out baby

You are ready (or so you think!), you can be sure your partner is ready, the birth plan has been memorised, all routes to the hospital have been checked and re-checked, the bag is in the boot, your work has been told about 'the date'. So what's missing? Where's the baby?

When expectant dads are first told of the expected date of delivery (EDD) they rarely consider that their offspring will not arrive according to the date inscribed on the kitchen calendar.

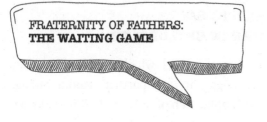

When we were told the EDD on our first, I recall saying: that's great, he will be a Taurus like his dad. Of course I got that one wrong. (I also assumed he was a boy!)

Tony, Dad of 2, West Meath

On our final scan, it was exciting to say to the receptionist that the next time she would see us would be when we'd had the baby; little did we know we would be back shortly afterwards in the same waiting room telling other expectant couples we were actually due last week!

William, Dad of 1, Dublin

We were given a date for our induction, which was great as we could get things ready at home first, though our unborn son had his own opinion on this and my wife went into labour on the way home from the clinic!

John, Dad of 3, Galway

A marathon runner knows that when he or she has passed the finish line, it is time to celebrate. In training for a marathon you are always fully aware that the course length is 26.2 miles, but what if after passing the finish line you were told you must a run a few more extra miles?

This analogy can be applied to expecting couples who have travelled beyond their date of delivery and are now treading the waters in no man's land. It is important that you both remain calm and focused. Reassure your partner that your baby will come out when he or she is good and ready. Preoccupation is the name of the game here, so try and keep busy. Why not consider the following alternative natural methods to induction?

Your partner should always consult with her obstetrician, GP or midwife if she is considering using any of these methods. Take note also that there is very little actual scientific evidence to support the effectiveness, or the safety, of any of the methods mentioned.

Sex: in extra time, are you kidding?

Sex is one of the most common methods practised to induce natural labour. Sexual intercourse can help to stimulate oxytocin – the hormone that causes contractions. Your semen also contains prostaglandins that can help soften the cervix in preparation for dilation. While sex during pregnancy will not harm your baby, it's best to refrain if your partner's waters have already broken.

The Man from Del Monte says 'pineapples'

Pineapple is considered to be a labour-inducing food because it contains the enzyme bromelain which is thought to help soften the cervix.

Nipple tweaking!

Gentle nipple stimulation can actually encourage oxytocin to be released into her body.

Homeopathy

Pulsatilla and caulophyllum are two commonly used homeopathic remedies used to encourage labour.

Going herbal

Blue cohosh and black cohosh are often referred to as being useful in bringing on labour. Raspberry leaf can also be taken as a tea or in tablet form. Raspberry leaves should not be used until the last two months of pregnancy because of their stimulating effect on the uterus. It is also effective in preparing and strengthening the uterus for a smoother birth. Herbals should only be used under professional guidance.

Fancy a curry?

Spicy food is often suggested as a means of bringing on labour; however, there is little evidence that this is actually the case. If your partner likes a good curry, then why not try this method. However, if she has a sensitive stomach, it may be better to give this one a miss!

Hands on

Essential therapeutic aromatherapy oils such as lavender and jasmine can be massaged gently on her abdomen or lower back area to promote healthy contractions.

Soak it up

Run her a bath adding a drop or two of clary sage essential oil which is thought to help reduce labour stress and may even stimulate uterine contractions.

Get out and walk

One of the best ways to stimulate contractions is to take a stroll (an amble, not a sprint!). The pressure of the baby's head pressing down on the cervix stimulates the release of oxytocin. Being upright encourages the baby to move downward onto the cervix, adopting the appropriate birthing position and engaging the head if they have not done so previously.

Ball play

A birthing ball is not only comforting on your partner's back and pelvis during the final stages of pregnancy but also provides a gentle way to get baby into the birthing position, encouraging the head to engage.

Not the Cooking Appliance!
Induction

When pregnancy passes the 40-week marker the notion of an induction is often tabled. It may also be on the cards if your partner's waters break and there is no sign of any contractions after 24 hours, if she has high blood pressure, diabetes or pre-eclampsia or if there are concerns regarding your baby's growth. If it is necessary to induce labour, your obstetrician or consultant will explain the options available to you. These will include:

Miyagi says: sweep the membranes

Your midwife or doctor will do an internal exam on your partner, sweeping their gloved finger around the inside of her cervix to loosen it from the membranes around your baby. This releases hormones called prostaglandins, which may lead to contractions. I have been told that it is 'quite' painful!

Softly, softly ...

If your partner does not go into labour following a membrane sweeping, she may be offered an induction using **prostaglandins**. Prostaglandins can be given as a tablet, gel or pessary and are inserted into her vagina. This helps soften the cervix so that it can open and contractions can commence. Most women will go into labour, although more than one dose may be required. After she has been given the pessary, the heartbeat of the baby will be monitored for a period to ensure no disturbance has been caused by the induction.

By hook or by crook

A long, thin, hook-like instrument is inserted and the amniotic sac is pierced and gently opened, starting labour off. Once the amniotic sac has been broken (i.e. waters have broken) your partner should begin having contractions. It doesn't always work, especially if the cervix isn't already open.

Just one drip

Syntocinon contains an artificial form of **oxytocin** – the hormone which helps the womb contract. The drip is put into her arm and gradually releases oxytocin, replicating the way in which it would have been produced if labour had started naturally.

Lights, Camera (Maybe?), Action ...
The delivery

There is no time throughout the pregnancy when a dad-to-be is in greater need of information than now. It would be an impossible task to present a 'blow-by-blow' account of how your delivery will unfold, as by now you will have learnt that the birth of your own baby will differ from that of the expectant couple in the neighbouring room.

However, you will have important questions and concerns and the following section is the 'daddy' of frequently asked questions for expectant fathers, and who better to answer them than a professional midwife who is currently conducting a study on first-time fatherhood.

Lorraine Andrews, Lecturer in Midwifery in the School of Nursing and Midwifery in Trinity College Dublin:

When do we leave for the hospital?

Some units in which you will have your baby recommend that you make your way there when your partner's contractions are one in ten (others say one in five) minutes apart (ie regular). If your partner is worried, scared, or if there is any bleeding or the membranes have ruptured, then you should make your way to the hospital immediately. To be absolutely sure, always phone the delivery ward and talk to one of the midwives about any concerns. If you live far away from the hospital then it is best to set out early.

What if my partner's waters break on the way or when we are at home?

Remain calm, use a towel for drying and comfort. If the situation permits, your partner can change her clothes if they are wet and wear a sanitary pad for the amniotic fluid (the water around the baby) that continues to drain. Once the waters are a clear colour then this is a good indication that the baby is OK. It is important to continue to make your way to the hospital to have your partner and baby assessed to ensure that everything is as it should be.

Where do I park when I arrive?

While you are at one of the antenatal visits or antenatal education classes it is a good idea to familiarise yourself with where to park your car when your partner goes into labour. Many men do a trial run to the hospital beforehand, for reassurance of the time it takes and where to park their car. It is a very good idea to bring plenty of euro coins with you when your partner goes into labour as this saves time and avoids stress looking for change for a parking meter.

What happens when we get inside?

When a woman is in labour she is brought with her partner to the delivery unit/ward. Here she is admitted by the midwife, labour is diagnosed, the baby's heartbeat is listened to, and vital signs are assessed.

What if a delivery suite is not available and my partner is ready to give birth?

A room will be made available near the delivery room and the equipment needed for delivery will be taken in there; often hospital units are set up for these scenarios.

Where do I stand or sit in the labour ward?

While your partner is in the labour ward, there is a chair for you; you can sit beside your partner throughout the whole labour. When your partner is in labour and both she and your baby are healthy and well, she may want to walk and move about and you can, and should, accompany her. Your partner can talk to the midwife about this and your midwife will let you know if this is possible and when to return to the labour ward for checking your partner's and your baby's health.

When it comes to the actual birth of the baby, the father generally stands up and supports his partner in her birthing position. Some men want to look down and watch the baby being born; others prefer to watch the birth of their baby from the top of the bed. Some women discuss with their partners beforehand their wishes on where they want their partner to stand when the baby is being born. While many men respect these wishes, some simply can't overcome their desire to see the full birth of their child.

Do all expectant dads attend the birth, and if I decide not to, where do I go during the labour and when will I be notified of the arrival?

Most fathers attend the birth of their child and for them this is a very rewarding experience to see their child come into the world. Often the mother is so tired and overwhelmed by the whole experience and it's terrific to have a dad to hold, love and get to know the baby. However, many fathers are very apprehensive about attending the birth of their child for many reasons, some being: 'Will I be of any use?' 'I will only get in the way.' 'I don't want to see my partner in pain.' 'I have a weak stomach.' It is best to discuss your apprehensions with your partner and verbalise how you feel about this, and you should do this at various times during the pregnancy.

Many men who are reluctant to attend the birth often feel pressurised by their partner or friends and relatives to attend. It is important to talk about this with your partner. You can also talk to the midwife about this at one of the antenatal visits or antenatal education classes, to see if they can help in some way to alleviate your anxieties. Should a father decide that he does not want to attend the birth, there is a waiting room for partners/birth partners near or in each of the labour wards. He can stay here until the baby's arrival when a midwife will bring him in to see his partner and baby when they're both ready. He can also give the midwife his mobile telephone number so they can phone him once the baby is born.

Am I allowed to speak with the midwife if I have my own concerns?

Yes, of course. It is good to get to know your midwife and talk to her/him and ask questions throughout the whole labour experience. This is a good way of involving yourself in the birthing process, but they will keep you involved as to what is happening. If a sensitive issue arises and you want to avoid raising your partner's concerns, you can excuse yourself and go and talk to the midwife separately, or the midwife in charge of the unit at that specific time. Bear in mind that asking questions when your partner is having a contraction probably isn't the best timing, as she needs to focus on getting through her pain!

What if I did not attend the antenatal education classes – will I be lost?

You don't have to go to antenatal education classes, but expectant fathers and mothers are invited and encouraged to go. Most men enjoy these classes as they gain more knowledge about the childbirth process. It also helps to familiarise them with the hospital and many get a tour of the delivery ward so that they can see what it is like, and this may alleviate their anxieties. Antenatal classes are also a very good forum to ask questions and listen to responses. Many men ask questions in these classes and their participation and questions are encouraged.

Is there ever a situation when I am asked to leave?

Very, very occasionally a partner may be asked to step outside for a few minutes. During labour and birth, emergency situations sometimes arise and the midwife and doctor may ask you to wait outside the labour ward room but will keep you fully informed about what is happening and why.

What if I feel faint? Has this ever occurred?

Yes, some men can feel faint and some men do faint but it's not that common. If you feel lightheaded, dizzy, sweaty or nauseous, at any stage, you should never be embarrassed to say it to the midwife, where she/he (or another midwife) will accompany you to get some fresh air, water and a place to sit down. The labour ward room can be warm, in anticipation of your baby's birth, and some men may faint because of the heat and because they have forgotten to eat and drink themselves.

Will we have the same midwife for the duration of the labour?

Depending on the hospital, midwives work either an 8- or a 12-hour shift. Most couples have the same midwife throughout the labour, but some may have another midwife looking after them, if a shift has ended or during meal breaks.

What else can I do for my partner in labour?

Many men ask what they can do to help when their partner is in labour. One of the important roles is just being there to provide moral support, comfort and reassurance. It is both an exciting and apprehensive time for the father to be, but his support is very important and is encouraged strongly. It is also a good idea to familiarise yourself with what is in the bag that the mother brings with her into the labour room, so that you can get whatever she needs and for the baby when he/she is born.

 iDad: **10 WAYS TO SUPPORT YOUR PARTNER DURING LABOUR:**

1. Hands on – many women find a massage helpful in easing their labour pains.

2. No. 1 Fan – encourage your partner; tell her she is doing great and that you are very proud of her.

3. Look at the size of that needle! Distract her during difficult contractions.

4. Speak up – remember you are her birth partner; it will be up to you to relay instructions in the birth plan to attending medical staff.

5. Take it like a man – some labouring women have a tendency to 'get it all out', and I don't just mean the baby; so take any insults on the chin, but be sure to apologise on her behalf to anyone else present.

6. Can you make me a sandwich, honey? Don't go making any requests of your partner. Ensure you look after yourself. Ask the midwife is there enough time to pop out for a sandwich.

7. Heavy breather – help your partner with her breathing techniques; believe me, it will do you the world of good also.

8. Get her into position – your partner may need to alternate birthing positions should she find one not working.

9. And we're off – you will be best placed to let your partner know what is happening down below.

10. This is your time to be an ARSE! Assist, Reassure, Support and Encourage ...

If it is a long labour and my partner does not wish for me to leave, can I bring my own refreshments in?

Many maternity units and hospitals allow you to eat (eg sandwiches and snacks) in the labour room; however, to be sure, it is best to ask this question at an antenatal visit or at the antenatal education classes. It is always possible for fathers to eat in the waiting room, or the café attached to some hospitals or a nearby restaurant.

As the labour ward temperature is a little higher than the home environment, it's important for the father to drink water or soft drinks, otherwise he will get very dehydrated and may even feel unwell, particularly if it's a long labour. The best advice is to eat a good meal before going into the hospital (if the situation permits and there is time) or early in labour and keep yourself well hydrated.

Who else is present at the birth?

Generally, a midwife stays with and cares for a woman throughout her labour. In maternity teaching hospitals it will be a student midwife who stays with and cares for a woman throughout her labour. However, the student midwife's care is overseen at all times by a qualified midwife. Should the labour overlap with another shift then a second midwife will take over the care. Once all is progressing normally that same midwife will deliver the baby. If there are any deviations from normal or complications, then an obstetrician will deliver the baby. The minimum number of people will be present in the delivery room. If your partner requires an epidural then an anaesthetist will be present to insert it. If the baby becomes distressed, a paediatrician will be present to care for the baby.

Most units only allow one support person/birthing partner (two in some places) to be with the woman during labour, eg her partner, mother, sister, friend or doula.

What equipment is used on my partner to monitor the baby?

The types of equipment that can be used during labour to monitor the baby's heartbeat are a fetal pinard, a Doptone and continuous electronic fetal monitoring. One or all of these devices are used to monitor the baby during labour. A fetal pinard is used to listen to the baby's heartbeat every 15 minutes, or more, throughout labour. This is like a small hand-held trumpet that is placed on your partner's abdomen. A Doptone is an electronic handheld device which helps the midwife to hear the heartbeat and thirdly, continuous electronic fetal monitoring is where the baby's heartbeat is listened to continuously throughout labour using an electronic recording machine.

What is 'Seeking Informed Consent'?

Informed consent can be either verbal or written; a woman needs to be informed of every procedure that is being undertaken in the delivery room. Written informed consent usually only pertains to a Caesarean section.

What if our obstetrician does not make the delivery?

When everything is progressing normally it is the midwife who delivers the baby, but should something go wrong, all the maternity hospitals/units will have highly qualified obstetricians present to assist with the birth, regardless of whether the couple have public or private healthcare cover. When a couple have decided to go for private care, the obstetrician will let the mother know beforehand if he/she cannot be present at the birth, for whatever reason. But they always appoint another consultant obstetrician to cover them while they are away, and this obstetrician attends the birth of the baby. If your obstetrician doesn't make the delivery, then you will still be well looked after.

I am very nervous about cutting the cord. Do all fathers do this?

You do not have to cut the cord. Some men find this is something they really want to do and for others it's not what they want to do at all. The reason why a midwife asks if the father wants to cut the cord is to involve him in the birthing process. The best advice I can give is that the father talks to the midwife about this during the first stage of labour, so that it will not come as a surprise to him if he is asked to cut the cord after the birth of the baby. Whatever the father decides to do, the midwife will respect his wishes as not all men want to do this. However, sometimes it is not possible for the father to cut their baby's cord, for example in an emergency situation.

Why does my baby look blue?

The baby can look blue as it's being born. Once delivered, it automatically has its first breath and pinks up quickly, but its extremities will be a little blue for 24 hours. Apart from that, the baby should never be blue.

What happens immediately after the birth?

During a normal delivery the baby is delivered onto the mother's abdomen and dried thoroughly. Then the baby is identified with two identity bracelets. Once the umbilical cord is cut, the midwife ensures the baby is thoroughly dry, then the baby is weighed, and a physical examination is conducted by the midwife for normality. Then the baby is wrapped in blankets, to keep him/her warm, and given to the father or mother to hold. Once the mother is comfortable, the couple are left to get to know their baby and they are offered a cup of tea! The couple and baby remain in the labour ward for about an hour after delivery. After this, they are transferred to the postnatal unit.

What is an Apgar Test?

The Apgar score is an assessment tool which is used to inform the medical care staff of the baby's well-being at one and five minutes after birth. The five criteria which are assessed using the Apgar score are the baby's colour, heartbeat, respiratory effort, muscle tone and response to stimuli.

Am I welcome to stay after the birth?

Yes, all fathers are very welcome to stay after the birth as this is a special time for the new family and most new dads spend much of their time with their partner and new baby in hospital. When there might be a problem staying on is when a woman delivers during the night and if she's in a ward with other mothers; the dad is encouraged to get some rest. It can be difficult to leave your loved ones, but then again most fathers appreciate the rest, and the time to break the good news to their family and friends.

They can go back in the next morning to see their partner and baby. Unfortunately, double beds have not yet been introduced into maternity hospitals in Ireland. Some maternity hospitals have an early discharge scheme, where the mother and baby can go home early once everything is well, and a team of midwives will visit the mother and baby in their home and provide care to them for a few days after delivery.

Can I film the birth? Or take photographs afterwards?

Often fathers do film the birth, but it's a good idea to check with your maternity hospital first or ask at your antenatal class. Photographs can be taken.

Do I have to leave the room to call family to tell them the news?

Most fathers make their phone calls to their immediate family in the delivery room once all is well with their partner and new baby.

When is my partner moved to her room? What if there are no beds available — what happens?

All going well, approximately one hour after the birth, the mother and baby are moved to their postnatal ward/room, depending on their cover plan for maternity care (public care, semi-private care or private care). Most maternity hospitals have separate rooms for those who wish to avail of private care, but this depends on how busy the hospital is at that time, and no one can envisage how busy their delivery time will be until it happens. If there is a room available, the woman and her baby are transferred straight away. If there isn't, she is transferred to a postnatal ward until a room becomes available.

How long must my partner stay in hospital after giving birth? Does it differ for a Caesarean delivery?

How long one stays in hospital after childbirth depends on the type of delivery and the general well-being of the mother and the baby. It also depends on the postnatal follow-up provided by the maternity hospital or unit. After a normal delivery, one can go home that same day, or the next day if the hospital provides an early discharge programme; if it doesn't, generally it's a 2–3-day stay in hospital.

Yes, it does differ for Caesarean sections where the mother and the baby are in hospital for 3–5 days afterwards.

They think it's all over ...

When he or she finally emerges, you stare in disbelief that this little messy bundle is yours. You continue to stare, however, at your baby and then at the midwife, searching for any sign of concern as fatherly instincts begin to kick in; fingers and toes are accounted for, both mum and baby are well, what do you mean it's a girl, I painted the room blue ... **Congratulations, you are a dad!**

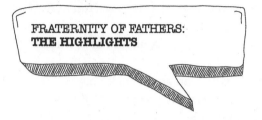

FRATERNITY OF FATHERS:
THE HIGHLIGHTS

I have never felt so terrified and helpless in all my life. The stark reality of the situation is that I was no use-nor-ornament in the delivery room, apart from being a familiar face for my wife. However, I would not have missed being there for anything as I had the privilege of seeing my son come into the world, take his first breath and pooh all over the place. It also raised my admiration and respect for women in general and my wife in particular onto a completely new level.

Adrian, Dad of 2, Meath

Childbirth is a strange experience. I can never know what it was like for my wife so I just had to be there for her, support in any way I could. She kept me close the whole time. I didn't go down the business end and I'm honestly not sure that's something I wanted to see. So I heard my girl before I ever saw her – like a little bird, she came out singing. Cooing. And then I saw her and I have never felt feelings so strong in my whole life. A love, a need to protect, just kicked in instantly. This was my girl. She had only just emerged into this world, but it's like we knew each other for ever.

The second time was odd in that the feelings were very different. Sure, that love and need to protect was there, but I didn't know this child at all – who is this little stranger? She was like a mystery! We've been getting to know each other ever since and, like a stranger being thrown into the mix, she has brought chaos but an unbelievable amount of fun and excitement.

Jason, Dad of 2, Dublin

I suddenly realised there was no going back now, my heart began to thump, I started to perspire, then the doubts kicked in – will I be a good dad, what if I lose my job, will he like me, will he be ok? I hope he's ok ... then you are handed your baby in a 'I believe this belongs to you' manner and everything you had been thinking of previously suddenly disappears ...

Mark, Dad of 1, Waterford

It was so fast. Two hours ago we were sitting in my mother's house going over baby names (again), now here I was about to cut the cord and my wife was asking had I put the alarm on!

John, Dad of 1, Donegal

We have two children; from these experiences I have three pieces of advice. First, it's a slow panic. Everything happens with manic action, but slow motion. Driving to the hospital, the long wait until your partner goes into labour and then the progress through the various stages of the labour. You keep yourself going on adrenaline. This means afterwards, you will be tired – obviously not as tired as your partner, but tired all the same. Be prepared for that.

Second, your partner goes through the real pain. But witnessing labour is perhaps the worst experience many normal people will go through. You're in the presence of someone you love going through slow-motion, excruciating suffering. You'll be the first of your new family to wish you could put yourself in the other person's place (but you won't be the last).

It doesn't get easier. On your second, you still have no idea what to do, where to stand, what to say. You still feel completely powerless as the professionals move fluidly in response to, or to trigger everything that happens. You still feel a very unexpected, new and potent form of love when it is all over.

Brendan, Dad of 2, Kildare

There are two great things about the childbirth – holding your new baby for the first time and the toast with butter your wife gets afterwards!

Paddy, Dad of 2, Dublin

I was made feel very welcome by the attending midwife. When she spoke about what was about to happen, she included me in the conversation; she made me feel very at ease which I was very grateful for.

Conor, Dad of 1, Dublin

What I was not prepared for was seeing my wife in such pain; it really disturbed me, and I felt useless and powerless to help. I could tell that she was only being brave for my sake as she saw I was on the edge. When she finally gave birth to our son I could have collapsed with exhaustion– sounds odd I know, but it was as if I was pushing with her the entire time. I have to say I was very proud of her.

Darren, Dad of 1, Cork

I was excited, elated, overjoyed – here was my baby girl in my arms, I was a daddy. I hadn't said much throughout the entire delivery to the attending staff; now you couldn't stop me, asking them where they were from, where they went to school, wasn't my daughter the cutest ...? My verbal diarrhoea didn't even stop when the obstetrician entered the room. I nearly shook off his hand after he congratulated us. He pulled a stool up, to finish up down below, and I continued rambling on and on, until my wife bellowed out: 'Ian, will you let him do his job? It'll be important to you that he puts everything back to where it was.' With that, he looked up and winked ...

Ian, Dad of 1, Cork

What is A LITTLE LIFETIME FOUNDATION?

Each year in Ireland approximately 500 babies die around the time of birth. As a result, a large number of parents, brothers and sisters, grandparents and friends are left bereaved.

A Little Lifetime Foundation (formerly **ISANDS**) is a registered charity which was set up in 1983 to provide information and support to bereaved parents and families. The charity produces and distributes a booklet called **A Little Lifetime** to all maternity hospitals and units in the country. This booklet has helpful and important information to help and support parents at the time they are told the news that their baby has died or is expected to die shortly after birth.

Their website also offers support and information not only for families facing or coping with this tragedy, but also for anyone who comes in contact with these families.

 For additional information log on to:
A Little Lifetime Foundation
www.alittlelifetime.ie

Afterbirth Antics
The third stage

The third stage of labour is all about pushing out the placenta. After the baby is born, your partner's body will continue to experience contractions. I know, has she not been through enough already? These contractions are not usually as painful as the previous ones. During this stage the placenta will separate from the wall of her uterus and begin to move down the birth canal. She will feel the urge to push and, in doing so, will be able to deliver the placenta with very little effort!

It is important to note that the placenta must be delivered intact. If any segments or pieces of placenta remain in her body, there is a chance that she could develop an infection, eg bleeding or uterine tenderness.

What happens to the placenta?

Nothing at all. Your baby's lifeline for the duration of the pregnancy will end up in medical waste. Doesn't sound right, I know, so perhaps you may wish to consider one of the following:

Eat it: Placentophagia is the practice of eating the placenta. It may be frozen or stored for later use, but in these instances, cooking or drying may be a better option than eating the meat raw, as infection may be possible after defrosting. Placenta is included in recipes for soup and lasagne. Many believe that eating the placenta can stem postpartum depression, replenish nutrients and increase milk production.

Asian cultures view the placenta as a life-giving force. It is often dried and added to specific placenta recipes.

Plant it: Many traditional societies bury the placenta and then plant a fruit tree over it – offering a living symbol of the new baby. Other cultures bury the placenta underneath an existing tree as a symbol of growth.

In Indonesia, the placenta is seen as the baby's twin and acts as the child's guardian angel throughout life. It is the father's responsibility to clean, wrap and bury the placenta on the day of the birth.

Whatever you decide to do, be sure to inform your attending midwife of your intentions or make specific reference to it in your birth plan.

Keep the Cord
Stem-cell collection

Collection of cord blood stem cells is a 'once in a lifetime opportunity' to help safeguard your child's future health. The procedure takes approximately 5 minutes and is carried out by your midwife, obstetrician or trained healthcare professional. It causes no harm to mother or baby. Stem cells are regarded as the 'building blocks' or master cells of the blood and immune system. Stem cells are 'unspecialised' cells and can develop into specialised cells such as red blood cells or other specific body tissue, to treat specific diseases. When collected, they provide a perfect lifetime match for that child.

 For an up-to-date list of diseases for which cord blood stem cells are used please visit: www.parentsguidecordblood.org

The Iceman Cometh
How are you **REALLY** feeling?

When a baby is born, a new dad is often overwhelmed with the realisation that this little baby boy, or girl, that he looks down upon is his: his to provide and care for, his to teach to shave, his to put through college, his to walk down the aisle. The great moment in question can see our new dad uncharacteristically shed tears of joy, and cries that can be heard throughout the entire maternity wing. Partners will look to the attending midwife and say, 'But he never cries!'

Alternatively, there are new dads who may feel no emotion whatsoever towards their new baby – will shed no tears and may appear to treat the entire situation as an everyday occurrence. If you happen to fall into this category, fear not, you are not on your way to becoming Ireland's worst dad. This is very normal. Rest assured, your moment of 'OMG I have a baby' will hit you later, and when it does you may have wished that you squeezed out a few tears back in the delivery ward!

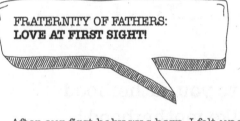

FRATERNITY OF FATHERS:
LOVE AT FIRST SIGHT!

After our first baby was born, I felt uneasy, very uncomfortable; I just wanted to go home as quickly as possible. I can remember sitting in bed watching telly, five minutes hadn't gone by when it hit me like a freight train. I cried the blooming house down. I felt so ashamed for making a quick exit earlier on and decided that I would never make the same mistake again.

Phillip, Dad of 4, Galway

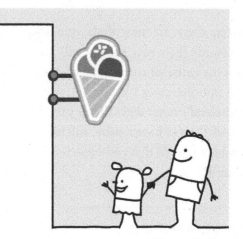

'I won't lie to you, fatherhood
isn't easy like motherhood.'

Homer Simpson

5 Surviving the First Six Weeks

We are family ...

You've just enjoyed two or three days' rest at home. It seems as if your partner has been away for a weekend with the 'girls' – the house is quiet, last night's takeaway pizza box lies open-mouthed on the floor with a few lonely bottle tops for company. What are you doing, man? GET MOVING! Your newborn baby and its mother are coming home!

The mobile will ring to tell you that your partner is being discharged. It will most likely be your partner on the other end of the line who has been sitting at the edge of her bed for the past few hours all packed up just waiting on the final nod from medical staff to say that all checks have been done and she is free to go home. Don't be surprised if she is a little miffed that you are not on the way up in the lift when she makes the call.

This is a very exciting and proud time for you. Bringing your baby home is the turning point for many new dads. After all, it is your chance to finally get off the sideline and start being dad. However, don't forget about mum and what she has just gone through. She will be dependent on you now, more than ever, for your full support. It's time for you to be a father to your family. Well nearly – there are a few things left to do before you leave home, so don't go putting the alarm on just yet.

iDad: **DOUBLE-CHECK**

Your local public health nurse is notified of your baby's birth and of your partner's discharge from care. She/he will make contact with your partner in the days following her discharge, to organise a visit to your home to offer support and information for the new mum. It is worth noting that should you or your partner have any concerns, the majority of maternity hospitals offer support for up to six weeks after your baby's birth.

You may also contact your GP or public health nurse for queries and services once discharged from the unit. Also, most units have a 24-hour emergency phone line.

Home Alone
The final checklist

The last thing your partner wants is to walk back into her home and see a pile of ironing or a kitchen full of dirty dishes. There are a few small duties that must be taken care of before you depart for the maternity hospital:

- When it comes to which chores to do, it's quite simple really. Your home should be in such a great condition that when your partner arrives in the door her first words should be 'Oh'. And while it's often encouraged to have a clean environment for a baby, the overpowering stench of detergent is not recommended.

- Do you have enough food in for a week? Quick and easy nutritious meals are essential. You will be tempted to reach for the takeaway menu on several occasions, but bear in mind that your partner will require healthy meals after being in hospital for a few days.

- Is the car seat installed correctly? If you are taking a taxi or if another party is collecting your partner and baby, do they have the necessary safety attachments?

- ⬠ Check that all nursery furniture and equipment are assembled in accordance with the instructions (and packaging has been removed).
- ⬠ Is the coming-home outfit laid out (the baby's, not yours)?
- ⬠ Check with your partner to see if she has sufficient post-natal supplies, eg maternity or breast pads.
- ⬠ Do you have the heat on (winter baby) or is the house aired out (summer baby)?
- ⬠ Have you shaved?

iDad: **MEALS ON WHEELS**

Many supermarket chains offer a delivery service across a full range of items from fresh vegetables to baby supplies. Items can be ordered online and delivered at a time that suits you. Furthermore, there are mobile applications which allow you to scan items wherever you are and add them to your basket in just one click.

Get Into Line
Managing visiting hours

You will find that once mum and baby are safely home the doorbell and phone will begin making more sounds than ever before, and instead of paying attention to your new family, you'll be shouting in from the kitchen, 'Is it one or two sugars, Mary?'

Having a family is all about adjustment, and this is especially important within the first weeks of the birth of your child. As your partner will be tired from the whole birthing process, it will be up to you to handle any 'appointments' to the house. You will need to be diplomatic in your approach. Slamming the door in your mother-in-law's face is a big no-no; an old school buddy who calls at 11pm with a bottle of whiskey to wet the baby's head should also be politely turned away (after bottle of whiskey is removed!).

Think carefully about rushing on to your Facebook page to announce the good news. This can often serve as an 'invitation' for pals to start calling when you need to be preparing the house for the arrival of your new baby. Use social media channels to delay visitors from calling if you must.

Family and friends may offer to do shopping, cooking or even some chores about the house. Don't be too hasty in blurting out that 'all is in hand'. Instead, be sure to take on help as is needed. After all, it will free you up to spend time with your partner and new baby or to get some much-needed rest.

 iDad: **BABYMOON**

The term 'babymoon' is often mentioned by travel companies as the last-ditch attempt by couples to take a quick break before their new baby enters the world. While this is a nice idea, which I'm sure would be welcomed by many couples, the term actually refers to the period immediately 'following' the birth when family and friends come together to help out around the house with chores, meals and caring for other children, giving you both the free time to bond with your new baby.

Having a baby is not only an exciting time for you both, but also for your families, especially for your partner's mother. Chances are that the new grandmother may be 'around' in the first few weeks, and this is not a bad thing (unless you have a rocky relationship with your MIL!). Having another close family member about who is also a mum not only alleviates some of the burden, but it can offer a degree of reassurance and support for your partner that any physical or emotional feelings she is experiencing are perfectly normal.

What is certainly not healthy is a 'know-it-all' who is constantly over your shoulder, telling you you're not feeding or winding correctly. Playing pass the parcel with your new baby should also be avoided. Of course, turning down requests 'to hold the baby' can be difficult, so if you feel that it is getting 'out of hand' take baby out of the room for a change or feed.

 iDad: **IT'S ALL GOING IMELDA MAY**

Mayhem, mayhem, mayhem ... Your lives are supposed to be all over the park in the first few weeks when you have a newborn at home. Wrecked, lost, confused, weepy, regretful, ashamed – and that's just the dads! Stop worrying about how things are right now. Everything 'will' settle down soon; you just have to find your feet. It'll take a little time, but as long as you support each other and look after your new baby as best you can that happy ending will come around before you can sing the theme tune to *Little House on the Prairie*.

BUMPEDIA: **THE HEEL-PRICK TEST**

The heel-prick test is a blood screening test that is performed on all newborn babies which is usually taken before your baby is one week old. This may entail a return visit to the maternity hospital if your partner has already been discharged; alternatively, a public health nurse may visit your home to conduct the test. As its name suggests, your baby's heel is pricked with a small needle, drops of blood are placed onto a collection card which is taken away and examined for any genetic disorders.

The reason for early screening is that should a genetic disorder be found it can be treated immediately.

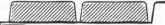

BUMPEDIA: **BABY BLUES**

After the birth of a baby up to 80 per cent of new mums suffer from a bout of the 'weepies', known as the 'baby blues', which comes on in the days that follow the birth and which can last from a few hours to a couple of days.

The physical exertion of childbirth and the sudden change in her hormone levels can be blamed for making our partners feel a little emotional, which is understandable really. It is up to you to reassure her that it is perfectly normal behaviour, that it will go away, and that you are proud of what she has just gone through.

Encourage your partner to 'have a good cry', ensure that she receives plenty of rest and make close family members aware of the situation, especially other mums, as they too can let her know that it is only a temporary situation and that there is nothing for her to be seriously concerned about.

Mothering Mum
Postnatal depression

It goes without saying that bringing a baby into the world, and into your life, can have a significant effect on a new mum (and dad – see below). Mum may find it difficult to adjust to this change as well as dealing with the daily demands a new baby can put on her. Of course a new baby is bound to make your partner tired and irritable and adjusting into a workable routine can take some time. However, for many new mums postnatal depression is a devastating reality that they suffer from without realising it, and so do not seek help.

PND can be mild, moderate or severe, and symptoms can begin suddenly after birth or appear steadily in the weeks or months during the first year after birth. The first step in being a supportive partner is in recognising your partner's symptoms:

- Tiredness
- Irritability
- Sadness
- Tearfulness
- Inadequacy
- Forgetfulness
- Nervousness
- Isolation
- No interest in food or sex

New dads must understand that it is a medical condition that their partner will recover from. It could take weeks; it could even take months, but your support at this difficult stage will help your partner make a more speedy recovery.

Postnatal Depression Ireland advises on how dads can help their partners who are suffering from PND by:

- Trying as a couple to go out without the children, but don't force her to do anything she doesn't feel ready for.
- Frequently assuring her that her illness is temporary and that she will get well.
- Encourage activity, even though she might resist, eg you might suggest going for a walk together.
- Trying to ensure that your partner gets enough food and rest.
- Giving her a massage. This will help her relax and restore her well-being.
- Reassuring her of your support and that you will not abandon her.
- Talking to her GP and public health nurse if you become concerned about her well-being.

Whatever you do, don't do the following as they can make the depression worse:

🗇 Leave her (alone) with the baby for too long.

🗇 Walk out on her, however difficult or impossible she is.

Postnatal depression threatens the mother's and father's health, marriage, friendship and career, as well as the baby's welfare. Dealing with issues on a day-to-day basis can be a special challenge for family and friends. With your support and patience, you can assist with the depressed mother's recovery.

 For additional information log on to Postnatal Depression Ireland at:
www.pnd.ie

BUMPEDIA: **SUDDEN INFANT DEATH SYNDROME (SIDS)**

Sudden infant death syndrome (SIDS), also known as cot death, occurs in infants under one year of age. SIDS is not just confined to cots but in fact relates to anywhere a baby may be sleeping. While the cause of SIDS is still unknown, there are ways in which you can reduce the risks of SIDS including:

🗇 Placing baby on their back to sleep.

🗇 Ensuring that baby does not become too hot.

🗇 Eliminating smoking from your household.

🗇 Keeping baby in a feet-to-foot position with head uncovered.

🗇 By never falling asleep with your baby in your bed if either of you are under the influence of alcohol or medication.

🗇 For the first six months, consider placing the cot in your own bedroom.

For additional information contact The National Sudden Infant Death Register:
www.firstlight.ie

SAD DAD
Male postnatal depression

The level of scepticism associated with male postnatal depression is undoubtedly attributed to its moniker ('Surely, PND is a hormone imbalance?'). However, up to one father in ten may suffer from it. A recent study highlighted in *The Journal of the American Medical Association* on the effects of 'Prenatal and Postpartum Depression' in fathers referenced 'paternal depression' as being a poorly misunderstood condition, receiving little attention from researchers or clinicians.

The birth of a new baby is a major landmark event in any couple's life; however, the reality of the situation can be somewhat different for new dads.

The change in lifestyle, the feeling of exclusion after the baby is born, the general apprehension of fatherhood, and, of course, the obvious demands and upheaval a newborn can bring can cause a great deal of stress for new fathers. Although expectant dads have the entire nine months to familiarise themselves with the notion of fatherhood, many feel that the situation is not 'actually' real until they are holding their baby for the first time.

While postnatal depression in mothers first came to light in the 1950s, it was not until very recently that medical professionals started applying the same diagnosis to fathers. But if postnatal depression is very much a 'hormonal' and psychological condition, what is it exactly that man can claim to possess?

Over-tiredness is a common foe of any new parent which can easily be written off as a result of sleepless nights. However, if this is accompanied by a change in eating pattern, insomnia or unexplainable irritation, paternal depression could be setting in.

Other common symptoms include: loss of libido, feelings of being overwhelmed, isolation and disconnection, the use of drugs or alcohol and submerging oneself in work as a part of the withdrawal. These symptoms are most prevalent in the first six months after a baby's birth.

A dad whose partner is suffering from PND is said to be at greater risk of developing depression in the postnatal period, with many female sufferers citing that their partners were showing similar symptoms to their own.

Historically men have been reluctant to talk about this type of depression, and statistics regarding paternal depression have only recently highlighted the problem.

The Eastern Virginia Medical School found that many new fathers experience postnatal depression, yet most cases go undetected and untreated according to the team behind the research. Based on 43 studies involving 28,004 parents from 16 different countries, including the UK and the US, the research team found that new fathers were generally happiest in the early weeks after the birth of their baby – with depression kicking in after three to six months – and that at least 10% and up to 25% had postnatal depression.

They called for doctors to watch out for symptoms of postnatal depression in men, as much as in women, and even suggested that new parents could be offered treatment as a couple. Other studies have suggested that the figure may be as high as 1 in 3 men experiencing depression during the antenatal and postnatal period.

A similar study led by Professor Irwin Nazareth, Director of the Medical Research Council general practice research framework, studied 86,957 families who received medical care between 1993 and 2007. They identified depression among fathers by analysing diagnoses of the condition and antidepressant prescriptions.

The researchers believed that the stresses of having a child triggered the depression – such as too little sleep, changed responsibilities and extra pressures being placed on the parents' relationship.

The influence of fathers during early childhood has probably been underestimated in the past. However, these findings indicate that paternal depression in fathers has a 'specific and persisting impact' on children's early behavioural and emotional development. The babies of depressed men are twice as likely to suffer from behavioural problems, including hyperactivity, as they grew older as opposed to those whose fathers are not depressed.

Today's society still dictates that men hide their emotions, quite often bottling things up in the hope that they will go away in time. The main reason that postnatal depression is lesser known is that men often find it difficult to talk about it, with some not realising that they are actually suffering from the condition.

We manage best in any new situation by being well prepared in advance of it. A new baby can be very tiring on new parents, so it is very important to ensure 'both' parties receive sufficient rest. This is also essential in the final few weeks of the last trimester. Alternating who takes care of baby on a particular night will also allow for a better night's sleep. Family and close friends are always at hand, so don't be reluctant to take up on the offer of a break. Consider talking to other dads who have survived the trials of early fatherhood. A little reassurance from other men will give you peace of mind that the early stages especially can be difficult and will help you feel less isolated.

Fathers should take solace in the fact that paternal depression is a common infliction, one that is perfectly normal. You should feel no shame in being overwhelmed in the first six months of baby's arrival.

If you are a new dad, bleary-eyed from sleep deprivation, and you are harbouring any of the symptoms mentioned above, then it is vital that you talk to your partner. Parenthood is all about negotiation and coming up with solutions as a couple.

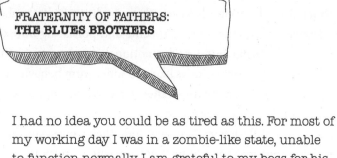

I had no idea you could be as tired as this. For most of my working day I was in a zombie-like state, unable to function normally. I am grateful to my boss for his support; the fact that he was a relatively new dad himself did help my situation. I suppose I was more of a spectator throughout the pregnancy so when the day finally arrived I was very much taken off guard.

Gerry, Dad of 1, Waterford

I can recall my wife telling her sister that I was a bit down for a while after our baby was born. Shortly afterwards, her sister rang me in work to berate me out of it, saying that didn't my wife have enough to worry about without looking after me as well? I have to say that I felt very ashamed. Is it no wonder that men remain mute when it comes to this subject?

Jonathan, Dad of 2, Roscommon

 iDad: **THE WAY IT WAS BEFORE**

A new baby is bound to bring some change to your life. It can be often difficult to find the time to be alone together, like it was before your baby came along. It is very normal for new dads to feel jealous of the attention that mum is giving the baby, with many feeling ignored in the first few months, and others, guilty for wanting it to be back to when it was just them and their partner.

These thoughts and feelings will pass, but it is imperative that you communicate with your partner how you feel. It is essential to your relationship that you establish time alone together, even if it's just a simple lunch date or walk in the park. Establishing 'you and me' time should commence from the very beginning. This way you not only have something to look forward to, but also that it becomes very much part of family life.

Continuing on with each other's own interests should also be encouraged, but again, play fair; this is an area that should be shared equally, and mum should not always be left holding the baby!

How to:
Change a nappy

As you take your first steps into parenthood one thing will become evident: that in the battle of the sexes, one will be victorious over the other at certain parenting tasks. When it comes to winding (more on that to come), my wife is Gina Ford (your better half will know who that is!) – she only has to look at the baby and it burps. I could spend hours rubbing our baby's back as if it was a genie's lamp, and it would take till the next feed to get the wind up, if at all! But when it comes to nappy changing, I am king. How do I know? Well my wife's nappies leak considerably more than mine (though admittedly she does change more than me!).

New dads seem to recoil at the thought of changing nappies; granted it's not pleasant, but like most things in life, with practice comes perfection. Nappy changing requires speed and concentration but above all preparation, so have your tool belt ready ...

The workstation

- Changing table, or

- A wipe-clean changing mat/clean towel (never change the baby directly on the floor)

- You must provide a safe haven so that baby cannot roll off. Do not leave a baby unattended!!!

The tools (Assemble everything you need first)

- Nappies, yes more than one; you just never know! (Disposable, terry or cloth)

- Safety pins or fasteners (for cloth nappies)

- Wet wipes or a bowl of warm water and some cotton balls/ wool

- Fresh baby clothes

- Nappy cream/barrier cream/petroleum jelly if your baby is prone to nappy rash

- Disposable nappy bag or nappy bin

- Item/toy to distract baby!

Before you start

Wash your hands. If you're in your suit from the office then you must be a pro or quite simply mad!

Here we go

1. Undo your baby's clothes and pull them up so they don't get soiled.

2. Un-stick the tabs of the nappy and fold them back on themselves (so they don't stick to your baby).

3. Undo the dirty nappy slowly (and quietly), wait for a moment, and if baby is smiling, you can be certain that a pee is going to occur — as babies often have a pee when the cold air hits their bits. I would strongly advise that if it's

a wee fella, you cover 'his' wee fella with a baby wipe to avoid any unnecessary showers!

4. Lift the baby 'gently' by the ankles, lifting the bottom and keeping the nappy in place use the front of nappy to wipe away any pooh. Fold the nappy in half underneath them just in case there is more to come!

5. Wipe the whole area using either warm water and cotton wool or wet wipes. For girls, always wipe from front to back to avoid infection; for boys, clean his scrotum and penis – never pull back his foreskin.

6. Lift both of your baby's legs off the mat to ensure bottom is fully clean, and remove dirty nappy.

7. Now, slide a clean nappy underneath. The clean nappy's top half (the half with the tabs) should go under your baby's rear, and the bottom half should come up between his legs (which should be spread as widely as is comfortable for your baby).

8. Pat dry (don't rub) if necessary with cotton wool or a tissue.

9. Leave the nappy open for a while to let air to baby's skin/to relieve nappy rash.

10. Cream is next, if needed. It's soothing and helps prevent nappy rash and infections. Apply sparingly.

11. Fasten the nappy at both sides with the tabs, making sure it's snug but not too tight. Ensure you can you slide a finger easily around the inside of the waistband.

iDad: **BRING ON THE CHANGES**

Frequent changing is the best way to avoid nappy rash. Let baby have a *Braveheart* moment and go commando of the nappy for short periods when possible; this allows air to circulate down below, reducing the soreness associated with nappy rash.

12. Reseal the tabs of the soiled nappy around its contents, put it in a disposable nappy bag, and place in the bin.

13. Dress your baby.

14. Wash your hands thoroughly.

15. Change suit!

iDad: **BITS AND BOBS**

For newborns, avoid covering the umbilical cord (you may need to turn the top part of the nappy down slightly to aid this). Also, if it's a boy, tuck his penis down to help prevent pee escaping.

The eco option

Non-disposable nappies are a popular alternative to the common disposable variety due to their eco-friendliness and all-round affordability, though they're not as convenient, one might say, as disposables. They come in two forms: pre-formed shape (usually with built-in fastenings) or flat, foldable terry cloths (which you fasten with a safety pin). Changing baby using either option is the same; the only difference is the way they are fastened. Obviously, you don't throw away non-disposable nappies!

BUMPEDIA: **MECONIUM**

In the days following the birth of your baby, he will pass some thick, green, tar-like stuff known as 'meconium' out of his bum. Meconium is a substance that lines your baby's intestines during the pregnancy, which is released in your baby's bowel movements after the birth. There is no need to be alarmed as this is a positive sign that all is well.

Changing a non-disposable fabric nappy

Follow the instructions as above, plus:

- Make sure the nappy is folded correctly before you begin. (If you're using a waterproof nappy wrap, insert the nappy into it first.)

- If you're using a disposable nappy liner, remember to put it on the nappy.

- When using safety pins, place two fingers under the fabric before inserting them. The safety pins should point away from your baby's navel.

- Check that waterproof pants don't irritate.

How to:
Wind a baby

Is he possessed? Should I call the doctor? This is usually a new dad's first reaction to seeing his baby with wind. It is an odd and worrying spectacle: the pulling up of legs, the flailing about of limbs, the crying, oh the crying ...

Assuming you have attended your antenatal appointments, you have more than likely touched on the area of how to wind your baby. You may have even taken this instruction for granted, believing that all it entailed was a bit of pat-patting and then burp – easy, now let's move on to something a little more serious for new dads like the lack of sleep! Your partner may have also received a head start with the bedside refresher course post-delivery on the best practice in winding – expertly given by her attending midwife or doula.

- But what exactly is wind?

- Why can't babies do it without any assistance in the first place?

- What are the best techniques?

- How long do you have to do it for?
- Are there any natural alternatives that help?

Wind is the swallowing of air by a baby while feeding, crying or breathing. The air fills your baby's tummy, which can make them feel uncomfortable and full up 'before' they have finished their feed. If feeds are taken too slowly or too quickly, the amount of air swallowed may increase causing discomfort (a lot of crying).

Techniques

- Over the shoulder: Hold your baby up against your shoulder so he's looking behind you and gently rub or pat his back.

- Sitting up: The commonest method. Sit your baby upright, supporting him with one hand on his chest, with your thumb and forefinger holding his chin. Lean him forward slightly and gently rub or pat his back.

- Across your lap: Place him face down on your lap. Hold him firmly with one hand and pat or rub his back gently with the other.

- Bicycle legs: Laying him down on his back and gently rotating his legs in a cycling motion. This approach is normally the 'when all else fails' method.

iDad: **TAKE COVER**

Before you start, you will need a burping cloth, eg muslin (and not a dirty tea-towel!) for your shoulder or across your lap, to catch any projectile spews or stealth-like dribbles!

Do not be too disheartened if a feed comes up – you will always think that the mess on the floor could re-fill the bottle, but it's never the case. However, if this becomes more frequent with each feed and you are concerned contact your GP.

Breaking the feed

Some babies are unable to take a whole feed in one go, especially in the early days, and parents have often found that breaking up the feed allows them to bring up wind. However, if stopping distresses your baby then it may be best to complete the feed and leave winding till the end. Interestingly, breastfed babies tend to have less of a problem with wind because their feeds are smaller, and they can control the flow of milk more easily.

Winding until the next feed!

You've passed the 20-minute mark and there is no sign. In fact, baby is now well and truly in the land of nod and there is no stirring him. The hardest wind to get up is always the one that relates to the 3am feed! If your baby isn't bringing up any wind after a 'few' minutes, don't keep trying to wind him – it may be that he doesn't have any to bring up, or it may be released later – at the other end.

Time is winding by

So, how long am I the wind instrument? This varies depending on the baby. Most babies begin to bring up their own wind unaided or stop having trouble with wind once they can sit up or when their digestive tracts mature.

Wind power

If you find that your baby is distressed or uncomfortable during/after feeds, then it may be a case of colic. Other factors to consider include the possibility that you may need to change formula or teats, or breastfeeding mums may also need to look at their own diet as a possible cause. There are natural alternatives and over-the-counter medicines available to assist with colic, but in all cases check with your GP first.

Again, if you are ever in doubt that something is wrong with your baby, contact your GP immediately.

iDad: **A DUMMY'S GUIDE TO SOOTHERS**

Soothers, pacifiers, dummies, whatever you choose to call them, you will find that two camps exist on their usefulness: those who cannot live with them and those who cannot live without them. The dummy debate has been raging in families for many years. They may well be the simplest tool to calm down a distressed baby, but studies have also shown that they can interfere with breastfeeding if a feeding pattern has not yet been established, hinder speech development and cause dental problems.

However, the most significant study of them all suggests that using a dummy to settle your baby to sleep, even for a nap, can reduce the risk of cot death.

Whichever camp you fall into, be aware that weaning a child off a soother is not as simple as taking candy from a baby!

How to:
Bathe a baby

Anything that involves a new baby, water and a petrified dad invariably spells out 'dadaster' – never has the theme tune from an iconic shark movie been more fitting: 'da-da, da-da, da-da, da-da ...'

But it doesn't have to be such a frightening prospect, as bathing your new baby presents the ideal opportunity for you to get in some quality bonding time, and as long as you are smiling, cooing away and having some fun, your baby will feel reassured that what is going on is perfectly normal. After all, they have only recently come from a cushioned sac of amniotic fluid.

The Three Ts of bathing a baby are:

Temperature:

The water should be warm not hot, and so too should be the place of bathing. There is no point taking your baby out of his warm cot, into an ice-cold room and then into warm water.

iDad: **THE HEAT IS ON**

There are certain parts of our body that are more sensitive to heat than others, the skin on our inner wrist for example is thinner and more sensitive to heat than the skin on our hands, so squirting baby's milk on our wrists will give a more accurate indication of the temperature. The traditional method of checking the **temperature** of a baby's bath with our elbows is another, as our elbows are particularly sensitive to heat.

Some babies may jolt at the first contact with the water and become distressed. If this happens, don't panic. Try introducing your baby to the water by gently rubbing them with a warm cloth first or scooping up some water in a cup and allowing it to trickle down on their feet or legs. Babies do not need to soak in a bath; a short, enjoyable experience, especially in the early days, is all that is needed.

Tools:

Have everything you need laid out first. If you forget an item, then you'll have to take baby out of the bath in order to retrieve it and this can be quite difficult to do when your baby is wet and slippery. Screaming down the stairs to your partner during *Eastenders* will go some way to shattering the bonding experience!

Checklist:

- A basin, plastic bathing tub, or sink.
- A few washcloths/sponges – preferably in different bright colours.
- Mild baby soap/cleanser.
- 'Baby' shampoo – use a small amount, not a bucket-load. We don't want to go testing that 'no more tears' theory too much.
- Cotton balls/wool.
- New babies often have dry, flaky or peeling skin, which is normal; however, a little lotion can often remedy this.
- Soft towel – ones with a hood are very useful to keep baby warm.
- A cup for scooping up water.
- A squeaky toy.

Technique:

Babies do not need to have a bath every day as this can dry out their skin; bathing two to three times a week is fine. You may find the following steps useful:

- When washing your baby, always think of the cleanest to dirtiest areas first; top to bottom is another way of looking at it.
- Wash your baby's eyes and navel with sterilised water and cotton ball/wool.

- Wash your baby's hair and scalp very gently, using soap or a baby shampoo. To prevent shampoo getting into the eyes, tip her head backward and place your hand over her forehead above the eyes; this way the water will drain down the side of her face.

- Babies who still have an umbilical cord stump, which usually falls off between seven and fourteen days after birth, should be washed down with a warm cloth; a baby is only ready for a tub bath (or sink) when the umbilical cord stump has fallen off and is free of infection.

- Keep at least one hand on your baby at all times and NEVER ever leave them unattended.

- When finished, pat your baby dry with a soft towel and dress in warm clothes. Don't forget the nappy!

iDad: GIVE ME SOME SKIN

Studies conducted by the University in Ramat-Gan in Israel suggest that, like women, new fathers exude hormones that strengthen their attachment to their infants.

Research discovered that a rise in the hormones prolactin and oxytocin, also known affectionately as the 'cuddle chemical', found in new dads has been linked to their ability to bond more effectively with their new baby. Hormone levels in new dads were tested in the first six months after their child's birth and a clear link was found between their ability to bond with their child and the higher levels of these hormones. The researchers suggested these hormones rewire men's brains in the months after becoming a dad, hence preparing them for fatherhood.

How to:
Stop a baby crying

Babies cry – it is their only method of communication. Not a pleasant sound, I will admit, but a fact nonetheless, and one that all new parents must accept from day one. Chances are you will find yourselves staring desperately at one another, waiting for one to step forward and finally say, 'I know what to do', but this rarely happens. In the same way that there is no cure for the everyday common cold, there is no secret method that can muffle a baby in full-on banshee mode. Start by eliminating the obvious: your baby may be hungry (even after a feed), may still have some trapped wind to get out or may need a nappy change. If your baby is just being 'a baby', then you may wish to try some of the following methods of calming your crying baby:

1. **Rock-a-bye-baby:** Hold baby close to you and rock/sway baby in your arms whilst moving. Rocking helps soothe agitated babies as it replicates the constant feeling of motion in the womb. Try rocking your baby in your arms, in their pram or crib. Be careful with rocking as this should not to be used as a method of getting baby off to sleep.

2. **Cuddling:** Don't think you are spoiling your baby if he needs lots of cuddling or enjoys being carried round.

3. **Place your baby** in the 'colic hold'. Lay your baby along your arm, with their head towards your elbow and their stomach in the palm of your hand. By lowering your arm, you can also ensure that the tummy is lower than the head to help wind escape.

4. **Swaddling:** Some babies feel happier firmly wrapped up as it makes them feel more secure.

5. **Fresh air:** Take them out for a walk in the fresh air, either in a baby carrier/sling or pram; the motion again will help to relax your baby and the exercise will be a welcome distraction for you.

6. Motor mouth: Try a car ride. Again, the movement is a big factor in soothing baby, but try not to become too reliant on this one and use only as a last resort.

7. Run a warm bath and get in with your baby: Warm water allows your baby to feel weight-free and to stretch more easily. The feel of skin-on-skin can often help to soothe a crying baby. If the crying doesn't afford you the opportunity to run a bath, try placing a warm, damp facecloth across their belly.

8. Hush little baby: Sing to your baby. It may at least drown out his cries for a while and help keep you calm. Let music also soothe your baby – that's why lullabies are so popular.

9. Try shushing: Loud shushing will often stop a baby in their tracks and so they will pause to listen. Though not an immediate remedy, this one may take quite a few choruses of shushes.

10. Cry it out: Try leaving them to cry for a 'few' minutes – some babies actually need to cry themselves to sleep.

11. White noise: Your baby can be calmed by 'white noise' – that is, noise that is continuous and uniform, such as a vacuum cleaner or hair dryer.

12. Baby massage: Babies like to be touched and stroked, so a massage is a great way to calm a distressed baby. Many babies love a gentle, rhythmic pat on their backs or bottoms.

13. Let your baby have something to suck on, eg the old reliable dummy/pacifier, a bottle, a teething toy, or daddy's (clean!) little finger.

14. Distraction: Sometimes a new activity, or dad jumping about, can be very helpful in turning a noisy baby into a quiet one. Try also looking out the window with baby facing outwards.

15. Take the nappy off: A common technique, similar to the freedom experienced in a warm bath, to stretch and kick-about, especially helpful if you suspect nappy rash.

With all of the above methods, be patient, as soothing a crying baby can take more than just a few minutes, and finding the right solution may require combining some of methods above.

If you are ever in doubt that something is wrong with your baby contact your GP immediately

BUMPEDIA: COLIC

Colic: widely defined as crying three hours a day for at least three days a week which 'usually' begins to ease off between three and five months of age.

Ronald G Barr developed **The Period of Purple Crying** for the National Center on Shaken Baby Syndrome, based on research of normal infant crying patterns. Parents who discovered the programme found that they finally had something to describe what they were going through, reporting that the word 'colic' was difficult to get a handle on.

The acronym **PURPLE** is used to describe specific characteristics of an infant's crying that allow parents know that what they are experiencing is indeed normal and, although frustrating, is simply a phase in their child's development that will pass.

There is a **PEAK** to the crying – baby cries more and more each week, until it reaches a peak at around 2 months of age, and then it decreases over the following months.

The crying is **UNEXPECTED** – you don't know when or where it will start or stop.

The child tends to **RESIST** soothing – no matter what you do, the baby doesn't stop crying.

The child may have a **PAIN-LIKE** face while crying – the baby may look like it is in pain, although it is not.

The crying may be very **LONG LASTING** – it can last as much as five hours a day or more.

The crying increases in the **EVENING** or late afternoon.

Wolverine Rocks!
Say no to rocking

I recall reading an interview with the Aussie actor Hugh Jackman in which he was asked what advice he would give to new dads. He referred to rocking your newborn to sleep as a big no-no, a bad habit, which for him lasted right up to when his daughter took her first steps!

Now I must confess, I too 'was' a member of 'The Rockers', couldn't help myself really. On hearing a stirring in the manger, I would dash like an Olympian, take babe in arms and kick off a rendition of Rock-a-bye-baby. I have to say that I was good at this; my daughter would be off to sleep before my wife could say, 'Will you get back into bed!' But there was another downside to being a 'rocker' – the system was not exclusively for night-settling; for each time my baby daughter had to go to bed she had to be rocked in my arms (and sung to!).

Going out for a 'rare' romantic meal did not mean services were suspended. Dressed to the nines, singing voice now low (in case the mother-in-law downstairs hears), baby asleep, out the door, mother-in-law smirking and pointing at the monitor. On return, into living room, hello mother-in-law and hello baby! As I said, I am the rocker; there are no substitutes.

It became hard for me to break the routine (or, as I saw it at the time, my own unique bond with my first born), but the fact of the matter was that after nearly a year I was beginning to conjure up images of doing this well into her teens and, on top of all that, we were expecting again and there was no way I was going to go down this same road again, sorry number 2!

So how did it come to an end? I first ceased the swaying, just held my baby in my arms but still sang. It did take longer for her to fall asleep, but it worked nonetheless. Then the singing was next to go after a few days. Of course, I would like to say case closed, but a few episodes still did occur now and again and a gentle rub on the side of the head replaced the arm boating method.

So take note: if you are a rocker (or intend to be!) and if you put your baby to bed and he or she cries, don't pick baby up. You can stay in the room so baby doesn't become distressed. Although most babies can be sleep-trained in three or four days, it may possibly take longer, especially if they are older. You must commit to sticking to a routine for at least a week, tantrums and lengthy crying spells included.

Gone with the Sleep
Surviving sleep deprivation

If new babies came with a health warning it would read: 'May Cause Sleep Disturbance.'

It's like this. Ask any other father what it was like in the first few weeks (or months!) when their new baby was home and you are likely to hear the following descriptions: hellish, like nothing I have ever experienced before, unbelievably stressful, I thought it would never end ...

Sleep deprivation can come as a big shock to new dads when the focus of their attention up to this point was getting everything organised for when baby comes home. You seldom consider what life will be like when your new baby is home, and you unknowingly overlook the demands that a new baby can have on you both. Sleep deprivation can have serious implications on your health and is said to be one of the main causes of postnatal depression in new dads.

For the majority of new parents things begin to settle down after a few weeks, when normal(ish!) sleep is resumed.

The following tips will help you cope better with the sleep deprivation:

R & R: Along with all the preparation that goes into getting things ready for the new arrival, new dads must ready themselves by banking plenty of rest beforehand, so early to bed in the run-up to baby's first appearance in the family homestead. This does not mean switching to watching the TV in bed!

Night on/Night off: Take it in turns so that one does more of the feeds over one day/night (but not all!). This will give you and your partner the opportunity to get a decent chunk of sleep within a given period. Try to get to bed shortly after the last feed in the evening.

Weekend pass: Most men have moved beyond the ages when they thump their chests and say, 'Me work, you feed.' However, it can be difficult for Irish fathers to be fully alert and productive in the workplace if they have had little or no sleep the previous night. This scenario can often cause a strain on new parents. Try to establish a routine that is fair and flexible but suits both parties.

Re-charge: Seek support from family and relatives, especially in the early days, be it to call round to allow you get out, or more importantly to take a nap. A twenty-minute shut-eye will do you the world of good. Accept that the housework may also take a backseat for a while and try and avoid being the 'we want to do it on our own' new parents. This principle seems to fall more on new parents of first-borns – believe me you'll learn your lesson by the time the second one comes around!

Me-time: Remember to take care of dad; a sluggish, ratty father is about as useful as a pram without wheels. Take yourself and baby out for a walk in the fresh air – this will give you both a better quality of sleep. Takeaways are often a new parent's best friend in the beginning. Do your best to avoid heavy starchy late-night eating and, instead, consider healthy snacks over regular periods and ensure you drink plenty of fluids (and not too much of the brand that gives you wings!). Consider taking a general multi-vitamin.

Sleep battles: Avoid unnecessary conflict. A common subject for arguments amongst new parents is the battle over who had the most sleep. Lack of sleep affects both parents. So if you or your partner had a difficult night, try and be supportive and arrange for them to get a nap when next possible.

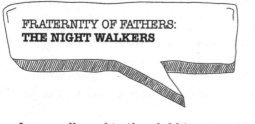

FRATERNITY OF FATHERS:
THE NIGHT WALKERS

I was well used to the clubbing circuit or going out to late-night gigs, coming in and having little sleep and then getting up for work. My friends who were dads would say to me just wait till baby comes home, it's completely different – they were right.

Simon, Dad of 1, Dublin

When my wife was expecting I would wake up several times at night after being kicked in the back by my unborn son who I'm sure was just having some fun disturbing the old man's sleep. In the morning my wife would say that 'he was very active all night'. For some reason the 'all' night part seemed to play on my mind in the months that followed – what if we were to have a baby who had the sleeping habits of Count Dracula? My theory was that an active baby in the womb at night was inevitably an active baby out of the womb at night – my theory was proven to be correct.

David, Dad of 3, Cork

My job meant that I was on the road during the week, which was really hard on my wife. I did make a point when I was home on the weekends that I slept in with our baby so she could get some rest. It also gave me the opportunity to keep up the bonding process with my son which I was afraid that I was missing out on during my weeks away.

Martin, Dad of 1, Galway

I can remember the lack of sleep with our first child, but when the second one came along a year and a half later it was worse. When my son was born we could sleep during the day when he slept, but now that we had a toddler to take care of as well, this no longer became possible and we were both exhausted. It made us buck up though and sort out a system; otherwise I don't know how we could have got through it.

Ian, Dad of 2, Dublin

iDad: **CLOSE ENCOUNTERS OF THE BABY KIND**

Numerous studies have highlighted the unique bond that is created between a new dad and his baby after the birth. That bond is formed by being in close proximity to your baby, be it through holding, cuddling or feeding. Baby carriers are not only a very practical parenting aid that helps nurture that special bond between a dad and his new baby but are also very useful in taking baby to places that a buggy cannot reach.

Admittedly, there are some who scream out, 'No way! Not me – they're just for those girlie types'. However, for you lads they are available in a variety of contemporary styles designed specifically with 'men' in mind, including a range of football club colours.

It's Breast to Bottle it ...
The methods of feeding
The breast formula: Breastfeeding

According to the World Health Organisation, breastfeeding provides young infants with the nutrients they need for healthy growth and development. I could continue on and fill the following pages with further facts, figures and an endless array of statistics to validate why it is that breast milk takes the gold medal, but this is a book for dads, and many dads will testify that when it comes to choosing which method to feed your baby, your partner will decide which is best for the baby and her. This, however, does not give you an excuse not to discuss the matter or seek out information should you have any concerns of your own.

For the most part, and in my research into the methods of feeding, it appears that our role arises post-decision. Firstly, it is in showing our support and encouragement with her decision and, secondly, it is in our participation with regard to the feeding or assisting with the feeding of your baby. While breastfeeding is natural, it is also a learned skill that can take a few weeks for your partner to master and for baby to get used to. It is in these first weeks that mum can often be tempted to give up. Your support is vital to helping her continue to breastfeed.

Tom Finn is a member of Friends of Breastfeeding, an organisation which works to ensure that women in Ireland achieve their desired breastfeeding experience. He has compiled a few useful tips below, drawn mostly from personal experience, which will help you support your breastfeeding partner:

- Do your homework and read up about breastfeeding beforehand.

- Encourage your partner to attend a local support group BEFORE baby is born. Other mums have a wealth of knowledge.

- Knowing how it 'works' is the most important factor. The more your baby suckles at the breast, the more milk will be made. Breastfeeding works by demand and supply. Instead of assuming that when your baby is feeding a lot that they may not be getting enough, know that the more they feed, the more milk there will be.

- Each mother's milk adapts to meet her baby's needs, so for the normal baby, there is no need to give water or anything else until after 6 months. For example, in warmer countries milk tends to be more liquid. Even if it becomes warmer for a few days, the milk adapts to that.

- Don't watch the clock. Time and frequency of feeds will change so don't be concerned. We don't eat at the same time every day so a baby doesn't need to either.

- Prepare meals and do the housework so your partner can concentrate on feeding your baby.

- Take the baby from mum between feeds to let her rest, and use this time to bond. I got so much enjoyment from my daughter at this stage.

- Encourage your partner, particularly when she is very tired or finding things difficult.

- Know that there is a breastfeeding solution for every breastfeeding problem.

- Be supportive when she starts to feed in public, or in front of family and friends. If you and your partner are both relaxed about it, others will most likely take your lead and behave normally.

- Be ready for baby blues! I thought it only happened to some women; apparently it happens to almost all of them. Roughly three days after giving birth, be ready to be particularly supportive. This can coincide with her milk coming in; it's a very emotional time.

- Breastfeeding only gets easier as time goes on.

◑ Breastfeeding is a personal decision. Some family and friends may encourage you to opt for bottle-feeding. Don't assume they know best; they may not. Be confident with your decision.

◑ Breastfeeding is free and very green. No bottles to be bought, so no washing up, no heating of bottles and no need to buy formula. Breastfeeding is carbon-neutral and also means more time to spend with your family.

◑ It is a proven fact that with your support, a breastfeeding mother is far more likely to have the breastfeeding experience she wants. Unfortunately, we live in a culture where breastfeeding is not always recognised for what it is – a normal way to feed a baby. If you embrace breastfeeding as part of your family's life, you will find things so much more relaxing and enjoyable for all involved.

iDad: **BOOB ENVY**

'I feel left out as I cannot feed our baby.' 'Is it right that I feel jealous of the bond my partner has with our baby?' 'I seem to be looking at my partner in a less sexual way.'

These feelings are very common for the novice dad who is new to breastfeeding. You should not feel ashamed or guilty in any way. Whilst we fully support and encourage our partners to breastfeed, at times certain thoughts can pop into the head that you feel you must suppress and not speak about openly. Now that you are parents you have a responsibility to your child and to each other to discuss all family concerns. Talk to your partner about expressing her milk. I'm sure she would welcome a break. However, it's important to note that breastfeeding must be well established before a bottle is introduced as some babies can get confused or develop a preference for the bottle. This is because the sucking action required to feed from a bottle is different to that used to feed from the breast.

There are many ways that dads can get involved, including winding during the feeds, changing, bathing and cuddling.

The seeing your partner 'in a different light' thing – c'mon, we are guys, this will pass and pass very quickly, I may add. Similarly the dads that say after witnessing the childbirth they would never consider going south again – seriously, how long did that last!

For further information on Breastfeeding log on to:
Friends of Breastfeeding www.friendsofbreastfeeding.ie
La Leche League of Ireland www.lalecheleagueireland.com
Cuidiu – The Irish Childbirth Trust www.cuidiu-ict.ie
Breastfeeding Support Network www.breastfeeding.ie

iDad: **A WEIGHTY ISSUE**

All newborns will lose some weight in the first week of their life. A 5 per cent weight loss is considered normal in the case of a formula-fed newborn, while a 7–10 per cent loss is normal for a breastfed baby. Most babies should return to their birthweight by day 10–14 of their life.

Get your teat into it: Bottle-feeding

There may be instances when breastfeeding is not on the cards: mum may be unable to breastfeed, or may have started out successfully and is unable to continue, or she has decided that bottle-feeding may be a more suitable option. There are a wide variety of formulas available on the market which contain all of the nutrients required for your baby's development.

Bottle-feeding (of any kind) provides a great opportunity for new dads to have some one-to-one time to bond with their baby. Usually, a feed by bottle will take up to twenty minutes, though it may be longer if your baby has difficulty sucking or swallowing or if the teat hole is too small or plugged up with formula. Alternating your holding position during a feed will give your arms a much-needed rest and go some way towards keeping baby more alert during the feed.

The inside scoop on preparing a bottle

1. Boil fresh tap water in a kettle (or covered saucepan).

2. When the water is boiled leave it to cool for 30 minutes.

3. Clean the work surface area well and wash your hands thoroughly with warm soapy water, drying with a clean towel afterwards.

4. Follow the manufacturer's direction when mixing formula.

5. Pour the amount of boiled water you require into a sterile bottle (see next page) and add the precise amount of formula. Adding too much or too little formula could make your baby ill.

6. Screw the bottle lid tightly and shake well (side-to-side) to mix the contents.

7. Always warm milk by placing the bottle in a bowl or cup of warm water. Be sure to test the milk on the inner part of your wrist to ensure temperature safety. The formula should be at least at room temperature to decrease any chance of stomach upset. Never heat a baby bottle in the microwave as the milk may be heated unevenly and burn your baby's throat.

8. Finding the right position for you and your baby is vital. Your baby's head should be higher than his body while he is feeding.

9. Make sure that the bottle's teat is full of milk and all the way in your baby's mouth.

10. Any formula remaining after a feed should be discarded as it's a potential breeding ground for bacteria.

 iDad: **ON THE ROAD**

Ready-to-feed milk is available in 200ml bottles/cartons and is considered the safest option when travelling with your baby. The milk is already sterile and once it is unopened it is not necessary to store it in a fridge. You can simply pour the milk into a sterile bottle and feed your baby.

The Importance of Being Earnest: Cleaning & sterilising

Cleaning and sterilising all feeding equipment is important as it removes any harmful bacteria that could make your baby sick. Bottles, teats and lids should be thoroughly cleaned in hot soapy water and rinsed well in clean water. A bottle/teat brush will clean any hard to reach places.

Steam

Steam is the most popular fast and effective method of sterilising feeding equipment. You can buy stand-alone sterilisers and microwave models that come with specific compartments that hold teats, lids and bottles separately. Tongs are usually provided to remove items.

Boiling water

Fill a large saucepan with tap water. Make sure feeding equipment is fully submerged and that there are no trapped air bubbles. Cover the saucepan, bring to the boil and boil for at least ten minutes. Keep the saucepan covered until you need to use the equipment.

Chemical steriliser

Baby bottles are sterilised using sterilising liquid or tablets (such as Milton). Make sure all equipment is fully covered by the liquid. Leave the equipment covered for thirty minutes (or as stated on the instructions), rinsing well with sterilised water when complete.

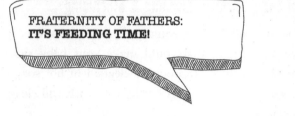

My wife was pretty sold on the breastfeeding idea and
it made perfect sense to me. Humans make milk for
humans. So I was all for it. And the midwives were also
pushing it really hard. When my daughter was born,
it turned out breastfeeding wasn't all that easy – she
wasn't taking to it. On her first night home, she was
screaming the house down with hunger and we had
no formula (because we were going to breastfeed, of
course!). A search for a 24-hour shop ensued and a
lesson learned. As it turned out, she got the hang of
breastfeeding, but what struck me was not just how
unprepared we were for any other option but how much
pressure there was to breastfeed. Thing is, it may not
have worked out that way and that's okay.

Jason, Dad of 2, Dublin

The day our daughter was born, the hospital midwife
warned us of the dangers of 'nipple confusion'. The
theory went like this: if you (the mother, obviously) are
trying to breastfeed and you give your new baby one
(just one!) bottle-feed, there's a chance that they will
prefer this easier method of milk delivery and reject
your milk production devices forthwith. We bought this
one for a while, but it turned out, in my daughter's case
at any rate, that there was no confusion. Our girl liked
milk – wherever she could get it! She could go from boob
to bottle, and back again, without seeming to be the

least bit concerned. Just so long as the milk flowed, no questions were asked.

John, Dad of 1, Roscommon

My wife was adamant, adamant that we were going to bottle-feed our new baby. I respected her decision but in no way did I exert any pressure on her not to breast feed. Bottle-feeding suited her/our situation as we both had jobs which required that we spend time away from home. What I did notice though was a Mrs Doyle (*Father Ted*) attitude when we started telling folks in the pregnancy that my wife had decided she was going to bottle-feed. It was constant: 'Go wan, go wan, go wan, you have to breastfeed', even in the seconds that followed a difficult labour. But even in my wife's weakened state she was determined and she pressed on with feeding our baby by bottle. Sometimes when we look back we get angry at the intrusion by others, even total strangers in an antenatal class, who felt that they could openly voice their opinions on my wife's decision to bottle-feed. Quite simply, it has worked for our family and we have no plans to change our minds when baby number 2 comes along.

Gavin, Dad of 1, Galway

I'm more pro-choice than pro-breast or pro-bottle, and though my partner tried her very best to breastfeed, it sadly didn't work out. Having said this, I don't envy being any woman who decides early on in the pregnancy that she wants to bottle-feed – talk about a cold reception. It surprises me really the level of contempt there is between the two camps; it's like United and City on Derby day – except for nine months and beyond!

Martin, Dad of 1, Limerick

We bottle-fed. Not so much because we were lazy ne'er do wells, nor because my wife had some kind of breastfeeding equivalent of 'too posh to push'. She just had huge difficulty with it. With both our children (and she tried diligently with both), it just didn't work out. I could explain why, but the description would be of such technical detail and complexity, you couldn't possibly follow it. This is because I cannot explain it – I am a Dad, a Male. The core of any advice I give to Dads-to-be is this: You Do Not Know – You Do Not Understand. The best you can offer your partner is *empathy*. You must be willing to listen and try to understand the situation. You cannot possibly fathom the guilt, pain, perhaps even depression, that your wife will go through if she cannot breastfeed – the best you can do is try to understand that this is the situation and you need to support her.

Brendan, Dad of 2, Kildare

 iDad: **SAFE & SOUND**

1. Do not leave your baby alone on a raised surface of any kind as they could roll off or topple over, eg changing mat/table, bed or bouncer.

2. Keep pets at bay.

3. Check that smoke alarms are in working order and avoid taking your baby into smoking environments.

4. Install fire guards and carbon monoxide detectors in the home.

5. Always strap your infant into a feeding chair, bouncer and pram.

6. Use suitable safety-checked baby toys only.

7. Keep small objects out of baby's way.

8. Never drink hot liquids near your baby.

9. For newborn babies the safest approach is to keep them out of direct sunlight. Put your baby in a stroller with a canopy, use an umbrella, or stay in the shade. Check the suitability of sun-block products before applying to your baby.

10. Make sure crib/cot mobiles and blind pulls are high enough that baby cannot pull them down.

Game on, Dad
Video games & fatherhood

As a new responsibility arrives in the form of that squalling bundle of joy, it is easy to lose parts of yourself. **Steve Boyd**, a veteran of the video game industry and self-proclaimed sleepless dad, gives his tips on balancing a newborn in one hand and a games controller in the other.

I am here to tell you, my gaming brethren, that gaining a child does not mean you have to pack away your PlayStation or X-Box, it just means that your gaming must adapt to the new situation.

When my boy arrived two years ago, we were on the cusp of a new Golden Age for gaming. Triple A, high quality titles seemed to be arriving every other week, but a lot of those were not exactly 'family friendly'.

They say that children pick up on things from an early age, so it is simply a matter of planning your sessions with your favourite shooter, or other genre, for when the little lady or fella is tucked into bed.

You do have new commitments now but, with a little foresight and planning, you can enjoy the wide world of video games and still be a responsible father.

- Arrange with your partner for a few evenings a week that you can set aside to pursue your hobby.

- They say that when the baby sleeps, you sleep. I say that when the baby sleeps, daddy can play! If the little one is going for a nap, you can pick up the controller and enjoy a half hour or so of your favourite title. Modern shooters have a multiplayer element that will give you a map or two in that time. Sports games and platformers are mostly designed in chunks of half an hour to an hour, and these can be enjoyed during Playnap periods as well.

◻ For the ardent MMO player, raiding is not a thing of the past. My guild is mostly made up of parents, old and new. Our guild (or clan or league) was especially designed for those with parental responsibilities. Two of our longest standing members have three kids and they use this as their escape from the pressures of everyday life together. Joining a group like this will give you not only someone to play with but someone who has been through the new parent thing before. They can advise on what you're going through as well as help you level up!

◻ Tailor your choices in games. There are a lot of games out there that are labelled as 'For Kids'. This normally means that they have cartoony graphics and little or no violence. Why not try those out? In my experience the gameplay and design of these games can be as good, if not better, than a lot of the more 'adult' games out there.

◻ Join the community! There are a lot of websites and forums out there that cater to you and others in the same situation. Being a gamer does not (always) carry the same stigma it used to. Check out the communities of gaming parents that are online. I have made many new friends through these avenues and you can too.

In short, being a dad does not mean you cannot be a gamer anymore! You just need to be a different type of gamer. It won't be long before that little one is holding a controller, or mouse, beside you anyway, so you'll need to stay in practice!

iDad: **ESTABLISHING A ROUTINE**

The concept of routine is not new to the parenting world. In fact there are hundreds of titles on the subject available in your bookstore or online which all focus on a similar premise regarding the feeding and sleeping patterns of babies. Getting your baby into a routine can be difficult in the beginning, especially as these unpredictable little creatures tend to make all the rules when it comes to feeding and napping.

Developing a schedule for your baby will not only provide him with a sense of security but will also give you both the opportunity to organise and plan yourselves in accordance with the schedule allowing you some free time to relax or take up those interests again that you may have had on hold in the past few weeks. It is important, however, to be flexible as we are talking about a baby after all.

Should you, or your partner, become concerned that your baby is not getting sufficient nutrition, or rest, from the new routine it is important that you consult with your public health nurse or GP before continuing.

Left Holding the Baby
Going back to work

It can be very difficult on new fathers to return to work after the birth of their baby. Fathers can often feel overwhelmed and, in fact, resentful at having to leave their partner to fend for themselves. Fathers must find it in themselves to make the best of the situation and to continue to show their partners the necessary support after putting in a full day's work.

Undeniably new mums will have feelings of their own, most likely that of isolation, the feeling of being 'left holding the baby' without adult company. They will often look to dad to take over when he arrives home in the evening which can cause a strain on the best of relationships. It is imperative that you communicate with one another and create a plan that gives both of you a break to recharge for what may be a broken night's sleep.

Where possible you may also wish to consider taking extra time off from work after your baby is born or make arrangements with a family member to call in to your partner so as she can have a rest of her own.

Relight the Fires
Sex after birth

You may feel that you have served your time over the past nine months with the notable absence of sexual relations. You have been consistently supportive and naturally sympathetic to her predicament, but surely now that the baby has arrived you can resume where you left off?

Stop the press my fellow man, there is a lot more to consider now than before. First off, let's dispense with the gory details as quickly as possible. Your partner has just given birth to a living being the size of a watermelon, and she may have also suffered a tear in the very place that you are eager to do business in, which needs time to heal, I might add. Her hormone levels are still off course; she may also be self-conscious about her post-pregnancy body, but most importantly she is likely to be exhausted and overwhelmed from the birth so at least let her unpack her hospital bag before you decide to raise the matter again!

Your enthusiasm is to be commended especially if you were in attendance at the birth – front row that is, and not in the safety zone adjacent to her head – as a high percentage of men find it difficult to re-engage in sexual activity with their partners after witnessing the delivery. Furthermore, the impending sleepless nights and the new resident in the bedroom can often quash any sort of bump-bump, so sex may be the last thing on either of your minds when you go to bed.

In normal circumstances a woman shouldn't consider having sex until after her postnatal check-up which usually takes place about six weeks after the birth. However, your partner will be the best judge in knowing when her body is fit and ready to start having sex again. Your role in all of this is to be patient and supportive – look at it as foreplay!

When the time comes, take it slowly and gently. You may also wish to consider using a form of lubrication. Handle her breasts with care, especially if she is breastfeeding – and not at the same time; that would just be weird! Speaking of which, it is perfectly normal to continue making love in the same room as your baby, though if you plan to wander down the tantric road you may feel more comfortable in another room.

 WHAT THE EXPERT SAYS:
POST-PREGNANCY SEX

The more couples continue to have sexual intimacy throughout pregnancy, the better their chances of reconnecting, so post-pregnancy efforts need to start in the nine months before delivery. Once the baby is here, couples should continue to communicate about their feelings around intimacy and ease into action, still recognising that supportive touch is going to be necessary for those times they can't – or aren't in the mood to – get all over each other. They should also plan to go on regular dates, leaving the baby with another caregiver, as happy parents make for a happy family and it's essential that they have private time together.

Dr Yvonne K Fulbright is a sexologist, sex columnist for *Cosmopolitan* and co-author of *Your Orgasmic Pregnancy: Little Sex Secrets Every Hot Mama Should Know.*

When Sex Can Mean More Babies!
The dad's guide to contraception

It is important to note that it is possible to become pregnant again very soon after having a baby, after 21 days in fact, and many unplanned pregnancies can actually occur in the first few months after childbirth. Being aware of all the available methods of contraception, especially those that affect you, means that you can contribute more to that decision as a couple.

No sex please, we're parents — abstinence

Yes, I'm serious. In plain speak: no sex equals no baby. Though, this is more suitable for the Zen Buddhist fathering types as it takes an insurmountable degree of willpower. There is no get-out clause here if you get my meaning, as even ejaculation without penetration can still lead to pregnancy.

On target — the menstrual cycle

Using the natural method of contraception involves your partner determining when she is most likely to get pregnant, and then avoiding sex during these times. By keeping a detailed record it tells her when she is most fertile. It has the advantage that no chemicals are used and also allows couples who want to get pregnant know when the best time to have sex is. Understandably, the figures for its effectiveness vary as it is depends on preciseness, mutual co-operation and determination on the part of both partners.

Building barriers — condoms, diaphragms & caps

Barrier methods include male and female condoms, diaphragms and caps. To avoid discomfort during intercourse, it is advised to use an additional lubricant with condoms to help make sex more comfortable for your partner. A diaphragm or cap is a flexible rubber or silicone dome which is inserted into the vagina before intercourse. A spermicide is often used with this method to destroy sperm.

Top of the charts — the pill and mini pill

Around since the 1960s, the pill is still the most popular form of female contraception. There are many pills available, most of which contain two different hormones (oestrogen and progestogen) and are taken daily at the around the same time for three weeks, followed by a week's pill-free interval. They are suitable for most women but should not be taken by breastfeeding mothers. Women over thirty-five should check with their GP first. The 'mini-pill', however, can be taken by women over thirty-five and breastfeeding mothers, as it only contains the one hormone – progestogen.

Stick it to her — the implant

An implant is a small device containing the female hormone progestogen, similar to a matchstick; it is placed under the skin on the inside of the upper arm. It involves a minor surgical procedure which can be performed by most GPs. The main advantage of the implant is its effectiveness (99 per cent) and the fact that once it is in place, you do not need to think of contraception for three years. However, the possible side effects for your partner may include irregular bleeding, weight gain and skin problems.

Getting the needle — injectable contraception

An injection that is usually given in the bottom, it gives your partner protection from getting pregnant for up to 12 weeks, but she must have regular shots in order to stay protected. It has a similar side effect profile to the implant, and some women also find that it takes some time for their fertility to return when they stop using it.

Mrs T — IUS

The intrauterine system (IUS) is a plastic T-shaped device that contains a progestogen hormone. It is inserted through the vagina into the womb usually by a GP. The IUS is a long-acting reversible contraceptive (LARC) which means that once it's in place, your partner does not have to think about contraception every day or each time you both have sex. An IUS can last up to five years and has 99 per cent effectiveness. Changes to your partner's periods are common; they may be lighter or disappear altogether.

Inside out — the patch and ring

Both of these methods contain similar hormones to the pill, have the same benefits and frequency of use but do not need to be taken daily. The contraceptive patch is stuck on to the skin, whilst the ring, a plastic see-through flexible device, sits inside the vagina for three weeks every month. As both contain the female hormone oestrogen, they are not a suitable method of contraception for breastfeeding women.

Naturally speaking — breastfeeding

Breastfeeding can act as a contraceptive when your partner is without a monthly menstrual period and is exclusively feeding a baby under six months old. Even if your partner is breastfeeding, it is recommended that she speak with her GP regarding other contraceptive options and the safety implications of each method.

Le snip — sterilisation

More than 99 per cent effective, male or female sterilisation may be appropriate when a couple decide to have no more children. In the case of female sterilisation the fallopian tubes are cut or blocked so the eggs cannot travel down to meet the sperm. A vasectomy, however, is said to be easier as female sterilisation can involve a hospital stay and the operation usually requires a general anaesthetic. A vasectomy works by preventing sperm from reaching the semen that is ejaculated during sex. It is usually considered to be a permanent form of contraception, although in some cases the procedure can be reversed. It is a quick and 'relatively' painless surgical procedure which is carried out under local anaesthetic.

Consult with your GP for further information and to discuss the suitability and side effects of each listed above.

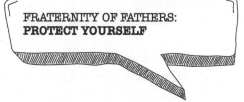

**FRATERNITY OF FATHERS:
PROTECT YOURSELF**

I was never really a fan of condoms. It felt like being a teenager again, but my wife was breastfeeding at the time and we both felt that this was the best and safest method which did not affect the breast milk in any way.

Tim, Dad of 2, Sligo

I think it became abstinence by accident. We were both so tired, it was the last thing on both our minds, and the topic of contraception didn't come up until well after our baby was in his own room and life began to return to normality. Sure, I missed the intimacy, but we were thankful for the rest.

Mark, Dad of 1, Dublin

I considered this to be joint decision and one I didn't want my wife to make on her own, so I accompanied her to our GP's office to discuss all the options. We felt the implant was best suited, so my wife made an appointment with the GP to return the following day for the procedure. Six months on, we are both happy. My wife is also thankful for the lighter periods!

Thomas, Dad of 2, Dublin

After everything my wife has gone through with the pregnancies we decided that I would have a vasectomy – it was the least I could do. The sex is still the same; in fact, I must admit it is a little more adventurous now. It really makes no physical difference whatsoever. The procedure itself did feel like I had been kicked in the groin, but the pain didn't last too long.

Richard, Dad of 4, Cork

For us, it boiled down to the fact that we were both simply too wrecked to do anything until one night when I jumped out of bed, thinking that I had slept through my turn to feed. My wife woke up, asking what was wrong; with all the noise I was creating I would wake up the baby – but wasn't that the point! No, before going to bed we had decided that we would see if our son would sleep through till the morning. We just couldn't get back to sleep from all the giggling we were doing and since we were both awake ... we cuddled! The next day my wife went online and searched a few forums on the methods of contraception. We deliberated over the various types and she decided to go back on the pill again since she had no issues before the pregnancy.

Gavin, Dad of 1, Waterford

We went down the road of natural family planning; my partner was breastfeeding and was determined that she did not want to take any chemical-induced method of contraception. Her periods were also very regular so she was able to easily chart her cycle.

Martin, Dad of 3, Galway

What's up, Doc?
The six-week check-up

Under the Maternity and Infant Care Scheme (the scheme that provides free antenatal and postnatal care), mother and baby are entitled to two visits to your family doctor (GP) after the baby is born. The first visit is when the baby is two weeks old, and the second is at six weeks.

The visit at two weeks is primarily to re-establish contact with your GP and to see how the mother and baby are getting on.

The six-week check-up represents the end of one journey and the start of another. This check-up is the final visit to your GP as part of routine pregnancy care, and is free under the Mother and Infant Scheme. But it's more than just health surveillance and promotion; it's about providing advice and support for families. It's a chance for parents to ask those burning questions that have been bothering them since the little one came along. Traditionally a check-up for baby and mum, many dads attend too and that adds to the value and the potential of the visit for all concerned. **Dr Tony Foley** explains what exactly happens during this consultation:

Firstly, the chat. You'll be given the chance to voice any concerns or worries you have. Your GP will enquire about how the delivery went and whether there were any problems for mum or baby. Questions will follow about hearing, vision and development: 'Does baby startle to a loud noise? Have you noticed baby fixing-on and following your face? Any little smiles yet?' The talk may then turn to feeding. Breastfeeding problems, formula-feeding issues and infantile colic are chief staples of conversation, while vomiting and dirty nappy dilemmas are debated. Upcoming planned baby vaccinations will be discussed and explained too.

Next, the baby's head-to-toe examination. Your GP will weigh your baby and measure his head circumference to monitor growth.

Attention will focus on examining your baby's heart, as sometimes murmurs, not evident at birth, will be detected around now. Lungs will be listened to also. Baby's hips will be examined to rule out any developmental problems and the groin pulses will be checked at the same time. Baby boys' testes will then be examined to make sure they have descended, as undescended testes is a common problem. Many rashes appear around this time and so a skin check will often be performed. Baby's eyes will be checked for a 'red-reflex' to ensure absence of congenital cataracts or the rare eye tumour, retinoblastoma. The examination may vary a little, depending on parental or doctor's concerns.

Now for mum's turn. The conversation will focus on how mum is recovering from the delivery. Issues raised will depend on the method of delivery. Wound pain or infection, mastitis, cracked nipples or engorgement, constipation and haemorrhoids often make for lively discussion. Your GP will be interested in how mum is feeling, as baby-blues and postnatal depression are common and seriously affect coping abilities and quality of life.

Postnatal depression may not be recognised by mum, hence the importance of partners being aware of the symptoms which may include low mood, tearfulness, disabling anxiety and lack of appetite, amongst others. The issue of contraception will then be raised – often giving rise to an incredulous response and jocular parental affirmation that a newborn is the most effective contraceptive known to mankind! Contraceptive decisions will depend upon whether mum is breastfeeding, whether the parents hope to have another baby in the near future and on past contraceptive successes (and failures). Mum's blood pressure will be checked, with further examination focusing on any particular problems raised.

Dads increasingly attend and participate in the six-week check-up. They express their views and worries too. Occasionally it may be dad's first time meeting the GP. This can be a great opportunity for him to forge a relationship with the family GP as baby's arrival undoubtedly prompts men to reflect on their own health and well-being. Paternal depression caused by the trials, tribulations and enforced insomnia of parenthood is an increasingly recognised condition affecting many men. While not routinely assessed, many GPs are cognisant of this fact and will enquire as to how dad is coping too.

And so the journey continues. The six-week check-up introduces the baby and newly formed family unit to the GP. It's a golden opportunity for all involved. After all, that's why we are privileged to call ourselves family practitioners.

Dad's the Final Word

Who is this guy with milk vomit down his shirt and a grand set of bags under his eyes?

No dad has ever said that the first six weeks were a walk in the park. If they did, then it's because they moved in Mary Poppins to take charge (or moved themselves out)!

Surviving the trials and tribulations of early fatherhood is about accepting that as time moves on life 'will' inevitably become a lot easier. Notwithstanding that adjustment, developing a manageable routine and ensuring that the channels of communication stay open with mum are all vital components during this testing period. Don't be afraid to get your hands dirty; believe me, when it comes to nappy changing, you will. You are also bound to make silly mistakes and be over-cautious, especially if it's your first – this comparable OCD behaviour tends to evaporate the more kids you add to the brood!

If you ever find yourself lost in babyland, another dad is only a buggy away. After all, we are a fraternity of fathers and we must look after one another.

Welcome to the club.

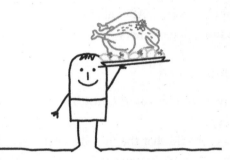

'The kind of man who thinks
that helping with the dishes
is beneath him will also
think that helping with the
baby is beneath him – he is
certainly not going to be a very
successful father.'

Eleanor Roosevelt

6 Men of the House
& the dad bloggers

According to the latest CSO figures, the vast majority of those who look after home/family are women, however the number of men who have adopted the same role has nearly doubled in the past 10 years up to 2016, rising from 4,900 to 9,200.

Role Reversal
The stay-at-home-dad

When first-time parents are expecting, they will undoubtedly discuss what happens when the baby arrives. Will Mum give up working to take care of the new baby? Can they afford the high cost of childcare? Or can they count on family or friends for help?

Nowadays, it is common practice for a couple to decide that Dad should stay at home. It may be that his partner has a greater salary, better opportunities when it comes to promotion, or it simply makes logistical sense. With a change in traditional roles, more Irish dads are seeking a 'hands-on' approach, thus resulting in the gradual fading away of the stigma associated with men who give up work to take care of their family.

Irish parents are now beginning to place an emphasis on the importance of quality family time with a healthy work-life balance, a shared parenting system which is very much prevalent in other European countries. This is quite evident when you consider the number of Irish men turning up at the school gates, attending parent-teacher conferences or taking the giant step in enrolling their children in their local playgroup.

Be it a decision arrived at voluntarily, or as a result of economic fallout, Irish dads are finding themselves in unchartered waters in one of the most challenging professions of their careers. Naturally they will have concerns: the loss of their identity, how they are viewed by their partners and indeed society, what happens when their children are in school full-time, and should the opportunity present itself to re-enter the workforce, will they actually wish to?

Being a stay-at-home dad is tough work: 'the hardest job I have ever done and one you don't get paid for', some men have reported. The role reversal has been a serious eye-opener for hordes of Irish men, quickly coming to terms with the fact that it doesn't get easier when you're at home. It can be frustrating and lonely at times, but the experience can be one that is extremely rewarding and fulfilling – that is, if you tackle it the right way.

10 Survival Tips for the Irish SAHD

1. Routine: the Holy Grail for the SAHD

By having a regular routine you and your children will come to understand what is going on on a daily basis, eg meal and bedtimes at regular times. A nap-time schedule offers a much-needed window to stop for a nice cuppa and a read of the paper.

Continue on as you did previously on a personal level with your morning ritual. If you were used to getting up at a certain time or shaving on a particular morning then maintain this routine. Often new SAHDs can slip into staying in bed for too long as well as getting lazy about their appearance.

2. Expectations and goals: from top to bottom

Keep your expectations low and flexible. Write down what needs to be done on a given day and don't set yourself unrealistic goals such as cleaning the entire house!

Trying to get everything done and accomplishing little can be very disheartening, especially when you are called on to entertain the little ones. Your partner will not expect everything done at once in the one day.

3. Fresh air: do it outdoors!

Being stuck in the house with children all day every day can cause a strain on any parent, so make an effort to get out of the house. A little fresh air and physical activity will make the day go by more quickly and help break up the routine; it may also contribute to a better night's sleep for all. If the weather's unfriendly, go for a drive – do not underestimate how excited children can get at the idea of going to the bottle bank!

4. Bad-sitters: here's the remote ...

It can be very tempting to leave on the TV or let your kids play video games so that you can grab some downtime, make a call, or do the housework, but use the 'bad-sitter' sparingly. Reading or painting at the kitchen table will offer your children far more mental stimulation.

5. Social interaction: my name is ...

One of the hardest parts of being a SAHD is the lack of daily adult company. Some dads feel a sense of isolation and, at times, even loneliness. It is therefore essential that you do your utmost to talk to people who are having the same experiences as you. Call up a friend and set a play-date, or join a local playgroup. Granted, it can be quite daunting to go into a predominantly female environment, such as parent and toddler groups. However, you will be pleasantly surprised with the reception you receive as many groups are very welcoming to dads. Check your local newspaper, supermarket noticeboards, and community centres for dad-only activities.

6. Join a club: man up

It is important for you to have your own interests/hobbies that don't relate to your children. Keep your mind active; this retains your identity and it also means that you will have something else to talk about with your partner and friends other than your children or the pile of ironing you have to get done.

There will be a variety of courses taking place in your locality at all times of the day. In addition to this, distance-learning courses are available online.

Many SAHDs miss the camaraderie that they once had in the workplace, so this might be a great time to get fit and join a gym, five-aside football or a running club.

7. Have fun: it may not last ...

It's not going to be easy but what is important is that you have fun with it, try to appreciate the time that you spend with the kids. Dads who do return, at a later stage, to 'employment' complain of being less happy in their new posts than they were at home raising the family – so enjoy the time with the kids when you have it.

8. Acceptance: when the 'H' is missing from 'SAHD'

It's OK to feel a bit reminiscent about life prior to 'house husbandry'. Accept that what you're doing is in the best interest of the family. Some dads have confessed to feeling a little less 'manly' and insecure in their new roles, afraid that their friends and even their partners would look at them differently. Putting your family first is the number-one commandment in raising a family. If you are feeling insecure, talk with your partner; never suppress any anxieties as doing so may result in ill-health including depression.

9. **Relationship: do you (still) think I'm sexy?**
It is not only important that you some get 'me-time' but
that you also set aside time to be with your partner. Organise
to get a babysitter in to mind the kids in the evening/during the
day on the weekend, so that you and your partner can get out
for a meal or go see a movie.

10. **Go freelance: open doors within the home**
It doesn't have to be all hoovering and homework; being at
home can also mean working from home. Home-based
franchise options can offer flexibility for the SAHD. The
web can also provide additional opportunities, eg blogging
(see below). Check with your local enterprise
board for 'Starting your own business courses' (see below).

Putting Word to Web

Blogs have been in existence on the web for many years. The word
stands for 'web log' and that is simply what they are – online diaries.
There is no level of skill or writing ability required in writing a blog.
However, there are tips that one can follow to ensure your blog is
engaging to visitors, which are highlighted below.

Stay-At-Home-Dad and dad blogger Jamie Harding provides
some 'words' of wisdom in getting started:

What are the different blog packages available?

There are a lot of good ones out there. Wordpress and Blogger are
both quite popular. I personally started with Blogger as it seemed the
easiest, and I wasn't very technically minded. It offers lots of different
options and layouts.

Are there certain rules to writing a good blog post?

Try not to bore your audience. Be funny. Write from your heart. If
you don't have anything to say, don't say it; you can always tell when
somebody is just blogging for the sake of it.

Do I have to show ads on my blog?

Nope, but if someone wants to pay you for essentially doing nothing, why not? It is all too easy to get precious about your work of art, but even William Shakespeare took the silver coin. An advert or two down the side of your blog isn't going to harm anybody. You can then spend the money on beer or on presents for the children.

Can I keep my blog private, just for family or friends?

Of course you can, but it's more fun, and probably more therapeutic, to keep it private from your friends and family, and public to the ... well, the public. Your brother-in-law getting too big for his boots? Tell the world about his collection of Barbie dolls he keeps in the garage. Change his name though, just in case!

What if I write something that is not politically correct — can I be arrested?

If you can't be arrested for being an incorrect politician, then how could you be arrested for not being politically correct? Stay clear of libel, racism – make that any '-isms' – and you should be OK.

Can I take images from the web to accompany my posts?

Your safest bet would be to use images from a royalty-free image site; there are enough of them out there. Outside of that, get imaginative with your smartphone and the plenty of cool apps that can make you look like a pro.

How can I let people know I'm blogging?

Facebook, Twitter, Instagram, Pinterest, Snapchat... Ignore that at times it's just a load of people talking about what they had for breakfast or what they saw somebody else having for breakfast. Social media serves as a great channel to meet other bloggers, publicise your blog, and find other like-minded dad bloggers.

What add-ons would you advise I install on my blog?

Presuming you took my advice on the previous page, include social media links/buttons. This will take people straight to your various social media pages where they can start following you. A 'subscribe by email' button is also quite good for making sure that your loyal followers get force-fed your product by email.

Do I have to allow comments?

Of course you don't, but you would be mad not to. They are the elixir of bloggers, the juice that keeps us blogging.

For additional information log on to:
www.wordpress.org
www.blogger.com
www.twitter.com
www.facebook.com
www.pinterest.com
www.instagram.com
www.snapchat.com

Daddy Dragon

There are 31 City and County Enterprise Boards located throughout the country that can offer support through business training courses, market research information, business-planning advice, access to business mentors and feasibility grants.

The Local Enterprise Office 10-Step Guide to Starting Your Own Business

Step 1: Business Idea

Have you got the right business skills? Who will buy your product or service? What is the benefit to them and how much will they pay?

Step 2: Market Research

From the outset, market research is essential in helping you to identify your target market and customers. It will also help you to identify your competitors and how to compete effectively. Research is also effective in assessing demand and establishing the real potential for your product or service.

Step 3: Business Requirements

Have you considered the best location for the business? What are your basic equipment requirements and costs? How many staff will you need to employ? Can your business idea benefit from new technologies?

Step 4: Investment Requirements

Identify all start-up and running costs associated with the business and the ways of financing your business venture. Seek financial support e.g. Banks, Credit Unions, Microfinance Ireland, family support, other non-bank finance.

Step 5: Marketing Strategy

Marketing your business idea is a fundamental aspect of starting up. Research the most cost effective methods of marketing your business.

Step 6: Sales Plan

How will you promote your product or service? Who and where is your target market (local, national, international)? What channels of distribution will be used? What is your selling price and break-even point?

Step 7: Legal Structure

What type of company will allow you to make the best decisions for your business? You could be a Sole trader, Partnership or Limited Company.

Step 8: Managing Risks

A new business can be exciting, however, it can also be risky. For some it means risking personal savings and secure employment.

Step 9: Avoiding Risks

Register your business name with the Companies Registration Office (CRO). Be aware of your tax obligations and register with your local revenue office. Other statutory obligations to consider include: employment rights legislation, trading licenses, planning permission, insurance, health & safety, patents, etc.

Step 10: Business Plan

Business Planning is fundamental to success in business – managing the company, generating sales and growing jobs. It is the key to getting things done and making things happen. The finished business plan can be used as an operating tool that will help you to make important decisions and manage your business effectively.

For additional information log on to:
www.localenterprise.ie
www.cro.ie
www.isme.ie
www.enterprise-ireland.com
www.revenue.ie

Chores Are All Done
Education & Innovation

Establishing a routine is the secret weapon for all stay-at-home-parents as it affords you the opportunity to do other things. However, the amount of time you have will depend on your own scenario and the age of your children. You may be a SAHD whose kids are currently in primary or secondary school and may find that you have time during the day to engage in other activities. Alternatively, if your children are not of school-going age and are at home with you during the day, it should not mean that you cannot engage in activities that broaden the mind or exercise the body. Admittedly, it may be difficult, but routine will be your saving grace.

With extracurricular activity comes a sense of personal fulfilment. You see yourself not only as the prime protector of house and home, and of all the little people that reside within, but also as your own self, someone who can talk about topics other than the three Cs: children, cooking and chores.

'Yes, Teacher'

More than 170,000 Irish adults each year participate in adult and community education programmes. You can be assured that one of the main reasons for the large numbers is due to the diversity of courses on offer. So, if you have ever had a penchant for getting under the bonnet of a classic automobile or you a feel a course of Tai Chi would help settle the nerves when junior throws a tantrum in the supermarket queue, fortunately Ireland is awash with a vast array of activities and learning opportunities that are most likely right on your doorstep.

Qualifax is your 'one-stop shop' which provides the most comprehensive information on further and higher education and training courses in Ireland. Qualifax has developed services to ensure that you have all the information you need to make informed choices about your education, training and career paths.

In the context of Qualifax, Lifelong Learning is the term used to cover part-time courses for adults. This can include short-term courses for leisure and hobbies, part-time courses leading to certification or continuing professional development courses. Attendance may be evening, part-time daytime or distance learning. The duration of the courses can vary from a few weeks to a year or more.

Qualifax is also part of Quality and Qualifications Ireland. The QQI Award is the quality-assured qualification awarded for further and higher education and training in Ireland. Learners receive a QQI award when they successfully complete a course at any of the 10 levels of the National Framework of Qualification (NFQ).

Spring Into Action

The springboard+ upskilling initiative in higher education offers free courses at certificate, degree and masters level leading to qualifications in areas where there are employment opportunities in the economy. Most Springboard+ courses are part-time, enabling you to keep social protection supports. In order to participate on a Springboard+ course you must meet the eligibility requirements, be resident in the state and also hold a valid PPSN.

 For additional information log on to:
www.qualifax.ie
www.springboardcourses.ie

Show Me the Money
What are your entitlements?

Whether you have made the decision to become a stay-at-home-dad due to financial reasons, have been made redundant or unemployed, or have simply decided that this is choice that is in the best interest of the family, the benefits, entitlements and tax breaks available to a stay-at-home-dad in Ireland are dependent on several factors, eg your partner's income, or if you are currently claiming social benefit.

The main benefits available to you and your family include:
Child benefit

Child Benefit is payable to the parents or guardians of children under 16 years of age. It is paid for children under 18 years of age if they are in full-time education, full-time training or have a disability and cannot support themselves. For twins, Child Benefit is paid at one and a half times the normal monthly rate for each child. For triplets and other multiple births, Child Benefit is paid at double the normal monthly rate for each child.

The Child Benefit scheme is run by the Department of Employment Affairs and Social Protection (DEASP).

If your baby is born in Ireland, when you register the birth of your baby the DEASP will begin a Child Benefit claim for your child and send you a partially completed claim form for your signature and payment details. If your child is not born in Ireland, or their birth is not registered within the required time (3 months), you must fill in Child Benefit (form CB1) and send it to the Child Benefit Section.

EU/EEA citizens and Swiss nationals working in Ireland satisfy the habitual residence condition for Child Benefit. If you are an EU/EEA citizen or a Swiss national and work in a country covered by EU Regulations, the country you work in usually pays Child Benefit even if your family is living in another country. However, if your children are living in another EU/EEA country you should still apply for any Family Benefits you are entitled to there.

The homemaker scheme

The Homemaker scheme was introduced to make it easier for those who provide full-time care for children or for an incapacitated person to qualify for a State Pension (Contributory).

One of the qualifying conditions for State Pension (Contributory) is that the person has a minimum yearly average number of contributions since entering social insurance to reaching pension age. The Homemakers scheme provides that contribution years spent working in the home while caring on a full-time basis for a child up to 12 years of age or an incapacitated person age 12 or over will be disregarded in calculating a person's yearly average number of contributions.

Working Family Payment (WFP)

WFP is a weekly tax-free payment available to employees with children. It gives extra financial support to people on low pay. You cannot qualify for WFP if you are only self-employed – you must be an employee to qualify.

You must have at least one child who normally lives with you or is financially supported by you. Your child must be under 18 years of age or between 18 and 22 years of age and in full-time education.

To qualify for WFP, your average weekly family income must be below a certain amount for your family size. The WFP you receive is 60% of the difference between your average weekly family income and the income limit which applies to your family.

The After-School Child Care Scheme (ASCC)

ASCC supports low-income people to return to work. The scheme provides subsidised after-school childcare places to people with children of primary school age who find employment, increase their employment or take up a place on an employment support scheme.

The subsidised after-school childcare places are provided by local childcare providers (both community and commercial). You pay your contribution directly to the childcare provider.

Affordable Childcare

As every parent knows, the cost of childcare is generally highest when children are under 3 years old – because more hours of care are needed and it is more expensive to provide quality childcare for very young children.

So, to help families meet that cost, the Government introduced childcare supports for children between the ages of 6 months and 36 months (or until the child qualifies for the free pre-school programme if that is later).

In addition, new increased childcare supports will be available to families on lower incomes who have children under 15 years old in Tusla-registered childcare.

Guardian's Payment

An orphan may get Guardian's Payment (Contributory) based on their parent's or step-parent's PRSI contributions. The guardian of the orphan(s) gets the payment. An orphan may get Guardian's Payment (Non-contributory), based on the orphan's means test. The guardian of the orphan(s) gets the payment.

The One-Parent Family Payment (OFP)

OFP is a means-tested payment for men and women who are bringing up a child – or children – without the support of a partner. A claimant must be separated, divorced, have a dissolved civil partnership, be widowed, a surviving civil partner, unmarried or be a prisoner's spouse, civil partner or cohabitant. To qualify for One-Parent Family Payment a person must also have main care and charge of child(ren) who is (are) residing with them, not be co-habiting with someone and have made efforts to seek maintenance from the other parent of the child.

Medical Card

A medical card allows the holder to receive certain health services free of charge. To qualify for a medical card your weekly income must be below a certain figure for your family size. Cash income, savings, investments and property (except for your own home) are taken into account in the means test. Unless you have a medical card, visits to GPs (family doctors) are not free. If you do not qualify for a medical card on income grounds, you may qualify for a GP Visit Card.

Under 6s GP Care

All children under 6 years of age living in Ireland are entitled to an Under-6s GP visit card. This covers:

- free GP visits
- assessments at age 2 and 5
- GP home visits
- out-of-hours urgent GP care
- care for children with asthma

Medication costs and hospital charges are not covered.

If your child or children have a medical card or GP Visit Card, they will automatically be registered for this scheme.

If your child or children do not have a Medical Card or GP Visit Card, you must register them for the scheme. You will need to provide your PPS number, child's PPS number & GP's name.

Family Income Supplement (FIS)

FIS is a weekly tax-free payment available to employees with children. It gives extra financial support to people on low pay engaged in full-time remunerative employment as employee(s). You must have at least one child who normally lives with you or is financially supported by you. Your child must be under 18 years of age or between 18 and 22 years of age and in full-time education.

Back-to-School Clothing and Footwear Allowance (BTSCFA)

BTSCFA is there to help you meet the cost of uniforms and footwear for children attending school. The scheme operates from 1 June to 30 September each year.

Back to Education Allowance (BTEA)

If you are unemployed, parenting alone or have a disability and are getting certain payments from the Department of Employment Affairs and Social Protection (DEASP), you may take part in a second-or third-level education course and get a Back to Education Allowance (BTEA).

Supplementary Welfare Allowance Scheme

Every habitually resident person in the State whose means are insufficient to meet his needs and the needs of his qualified adult or child(ren) shall be entitled to Supplementary Welfare Allowance.

Joint Tax Assessment

If only one spouse has taxable income and you decide to stay at home to take care of your children, then all tax credits may be given to the spouse with the income once you have informed the Revenue of the marriage by contacting your local tax office.

 For up-to-date information contact your local Citizens Information Centre or log on to:
www.citizensinformation.ie or www.revenue.ie

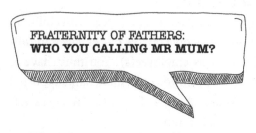

FRATERNITY OF FATHERS:
WHO YOU CALLING MR MUM?

Misadventures in the baby aisle

One month away from the birth of our first son, my wife and I were fretting over the dilemma that would soon show its face, childcare or not. The answer came quickly; the price of childcare would have cost nearly one of our salaries and was therefore not an option.

I was fully aware that as a SAHD there would be no breaks, no pay, no holidays and no sick days, but I embraced the role with the same zest I would apply to cashing in a winning lottery ticket. The learning curve was steep. The shock to the system was softened as my wife had the first few months off with maternity leave, but nothing prepared me for the challenge of flying solo. I discovered, by trial and error, that there is a world which runs parallel to the one we all know and love, that world is *the baby aisle*. In the baby aisle you have to learn quickly. You are forced to become proficient in lotions, potions, creams, medicines and all-in-one-sleep suits (with feet). There was nobody shadowing me with a gentle hand guiding me away from the 'juices which make them hyper'. I didn't know, for example, that nappies came in different categories and calibres.

Just like any job, though, I toughed it out, found my stride and got used to the routine. When I took on the role of a SAHD, I have to admit that I did fear being viewed by other blokes as a lesser male. I dreaded pushing the buggy past building sites and being judged. Surprisingly though, this type of scenario never materialised. The recession took care of most of the building sites, and upon hearing what I was doing, men, for the most part, expressed envy. The most interesting reactions I received were whilst I pushed my son on a swing in the local playground. I was asked whether I work as well as look after the kids and home and was also told that it's 'refreshing' to see a man do a woman's job. Both remarks came from women with children.

Our son turned 3 and with that the task eased as he became increasingly independent. Then one day my wife appears by my side and says, 'Look at this.' I turn to see her holding a pregnancy test kit ... indicating a positive result. Our second son is now 1 and providing me with all the challenges and utter delight I could ever ask for.

Nick, Dad of 2, Kildare

Taken for granted

When I was made redundant I knew that there would be no chance of securing another job any time soon. The past few years had rocketed by and included trips abroad, a company car and an expense account which included my domestic bills. This was all gone. Fortunately my wife was working. It's funny, I would often pass snide remarks about her profession, claiming my own was more important and that it paid the majority of the bills – now I was grateful that she continued on working. When we had the kids I encouraged her to give up work and stay at home, but she was adamant, determined to carve her own niche. Thank heavens for that.

Today sees me at home looking after our 1-year-old and 3-year-old. I must admit that it was difficult to begin with, but as the months passed I began calling my wife less during the day with silly problems. I have established a routine which works. I was never one for sitting down and watching TV, so I fill my days with kids' activities or preparing the meals. In the beginning I was paranoid that my wife would look at me differently and think me less of a man, but this was my own hang-up and I had to get over myself. I consider myself a strong person, so I could not care less what anybody else thinks of me and what I am doing. I am providing for the family in my own way.

Damien, Dad of 2, Dublin

Just not adding up

It suited our household that I become a stay-at-home-dad. It was me who presented the idea to my wife in the first place. I was sitting at the kitchen table one Saturday morning doing the bills when I came across the childcare and childminder fees. On the next line was a petrol debit. The childcare facility was a forty-mile, daily round-trip in a different direction to our workplace. It didn't make sense at all. When redundancy was offered, I grabbed it with both hands! I fill my days looking after the kids and doing the housework, but my mum drops by once or twice a week (to check on me I suppose) and I can get out for a run.

I also did a basic cookery course in my local community centre as cooking was my main weakness and there are only a few times that you can give your wife beans-à-la-toast when she comes in from a hard day at the office!

Sean, Dad of 3, Cork

The traveller

We had bought a new house in Cavan, a few years ago, and were enjoying life. The only real downside was that I had a daily commute to Dublin. I had to leave early and did not return until late in the evening. This all meant that I ended up being a weekend dad!

Each day I would sit at my desk and look at the family picture and ask myself: was it worth it? Not long after, this was answered for me. The company that I was working for went into receivership and I lost my job. My wife worked locally, so we had some income coming in. We had also put a little away for a rainy day, so at least we had that safety net. However, we had to take our twins out of daycare as we could no longer afford it. I am now the man-of-the-house; I see my kids every day and, if I am to be honest, I am happier for it. It can be very hard and desperately lonely at times, but you have to make sacrifices for your family. I know someday that the opportunity to work again will arise and it's that, more than anything else, I am dreading.

Richard, Dad of 2, Cavan

Only the lonely

After a few weeks as a house hubby, I started to miss the male banter that I had in the job working on the building sites. We were living a little out in the sticks so we had very few neighbours, never mind other stay-at-home-dads! One evening when my partner got home from work, I broke down, telling her that I was a bit depressed.

My partner recommended that I join the local footie club. I feel it is important that you don't get too bogged down with being a SAHD; it does take time to adjust and you will make mistakes, but as long as you don't bottle things up and find some time for yourself, you will be alright.

Jim, Dad of 2, Galway

Old-school dad

Are you kidding, me a stay-at-home-dad? I couldn't do it. This is what I thought when my missus mentioned the possibility of me looking after our new baby. But after we did the maths, it was the only real solution. Yes, I was worried what my mates would think, and my own dad was a bit of a man's man.

When the baby arrived I continued to work until my wife's maternity leave ended. I didn't run from any duties in the meantime; I changed, bathed and fed my son – a kind of dress rehearsal for when the day would come when I would take over completely. In the run-up I let all my mates know of the plans. Yes, there were jibes, but most of them were dads so it was more of a hats-off attitude to it. I'm 10 months in; there are moments, I will tell you, but he's doing great – like his daddy! I have also started back working on the weekends part-time to bring in some extra money, much to the delight of my own dad.

Ross, Dad of 1, Laois

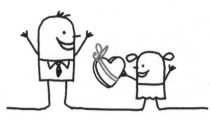

'Someday I may find my prince, but my father will always be King.'

A Daughter

7 Legal Issues

Everything you need to know but were afraid to ask ...

Paternity Leave & Benefit

In December 2017 The Department of Employment Affairs and Social Protection welcomed the uptake in Paternity Benefit since its introduction only 16 months previously. By the end of November 2017 some 29,700 fathers availed of the two weeks' payment, including 2,400 self-employed.

What is the connection between Paternity Leave and Paternity Benefit?

Similar to the Maternity Leave and Maternity Benefit schemes, you must have an entitlement to Paternity Leave granted by your employer (or yourself, if self-employed) before you can apply for Paternity Benefit.

What is Paternity Benefit?

Paternity Benefit is a payment made to a person who is on Paternity Leave from work and covered by social insurance (PRSI). It is available in respect of any child born or placed with their adoptive parents on or after 1 September 2016.

Paternity Benefit provides a weekly payment for two weeks to enable the parent to take this time off work.

Can I claim Paternity Benefit if I adopt a baby?
Yes, you can claim Paternity Benefit within 26 weeks of the date that the baby is placed with you and your spouse or partner, and you must provide confirmation of the date that the child was placed in your care.

What should I do now if I want to take the leave and avail of the benefit?
Notify your employer in good time and provide proof of the expected date of confinement of your spouse or partner. Ensure that you are in a position to make your application online at www.mywelfare.ie.

What supporting documentation do I require for my employer to apply for the Paternity Leave?
You are required to notify your employer at least four weeks in advance of taking your Paternity Leave and to provide proof of the expected date of confinement of your spouse or partner. In other words, you will be required to provide a certificate from your spouse/ partner's doctor confirming when your baby is due, or confirmation of the baby's birth where the leave is being applied for after the birth has occurred. In the case of an adoption, you must provide confirmation of the date of placement of your baby in your care.

What supporting documentation do I require to apply for the Paternity Benefit?
If you are employed, your employer must complete a form to certify that you are entitled to Paternity Leave for the dates provided. A form PB2: Employer Certificate (employee / PAYE applicant) is available for this purpose.

If you are self-employed, a doctor must certify the due date of your baby or the baby's date of birth. This is required to confirm that you are entitled to Paternity Leave. A form PB3: Doctors Certificate (self-employed applicants) is available for this purpose.

How will I be notified about the decision on my Paternity Benefit claim?

A decision on your claim and all correspondence relating to your claim will issue by e-mail to your 'MyWelfare' account.

How much is the benefit?

Paternity Benefit is currently payable at a minimum rate of €235 per week for two weeks.

Can I split the period and take separate weeks?

No. The full period must be taken in one block.

Will my employer pay me while I'm on Paternity Leave?

Some employers will continue to pay an employee while the employee is on Paternity Leave. In such cases, the employer will require the employee to have any Paternity Benefit paid to them. You should check your contract of employment to see what applies to you.

Can Paternity Benefit be claimed by men only?

Paternity Benefit can be claimed by the spouse, cohabitant or civil partner of the mother, regardless of gender, or by the spouse, cohabitant or civil partner of the adopting mother, or by the spouse, cohabitant or civil partner of a sole male adopter.

Provision is also made in the legislation that Paternity Benefit can be paid to the father of the child in cases where the father is not a spouse, cohabitant or civil partner of the child's mother.

We are two recently married men and I'm adopting my husband's son, who is seven. Am I entitled to Paternity Benefit? (My husband already took adoptive leave as a sole male adopter.)

Yes, but the Paternity Benefit must start within 26 weeks from the day of placement.

How is Paternity Benefit paid?

Paternity Benefit can be paid in two ways: by electronic fund transfer (EFT) into your nominated bank account or building society; or mandated to your employer's account where your employer continues to pay your wage while you are on Paternity Leave.

Is my Paternity Benefit subject to PRSI?

Paternity Benefit is not subject to PRSI. If you choose to have your Benefit paid to your employer, who then continues to pay your normal weekly wage, you may be entitled to a PRSI refund. You should complete the Refund of PRSI Contributions Application which can be accessed online at www.welfare.ie.

Is my Paternity Benefit taxable?

Paternity Benefit (including any increases for adult and child dependents) is reckonable for income tax purposes.

How do I qualify?

In order to qualify, you must be in employment or self-employment and satisfy certain PRSI conditions. The PRSI classes that count for Paternity Benefit are A, E, H and S (self-employed). Paternity Benefit is not payable to serving members of the Defence Forces who pay PRSI at Class H.

In the case of an employee:

⊘ At least 39 weeks' PRSI contributions paid in the 12-month period before the first day of your Paternity Benefit and

⊘ At least 39 weeks' PRSI paid since first starting work and at least 39 weeks' PRSI paid or credited in the relevant tax year or in the tax year immediately following the relevant tax year or

⊘ At least 26 weeks' PRSI paid in the relevant tax year and at least 26 weeks' PRSI paid in the tax year immediately before the relevant tax year.

If you do not meet these PRSI conditions and you were in insurable self-employment before starting insurable employment as an employee, you may use your PRSI contributions (Class S) in that self-employment to qualify for Paternity Benefit – see PRSI conditions for self-employed people below.

You are awarded credited contributions or credits automatically when you are getting Paternity Benefit. Credits are awarded at the same rate as your last paid contribution. These credits help protect your future entitlement to social welfare benefits and pensions.

Periods of insurance in another EU member state may be taken into account to meet the PRSI contribution conditions. The last week of insurance must be paid in Ireland.

In the case of a person in insurable self-employment, you must have:

- 52 PRSI contributions paid at Class S in the relevant tax year or
- 52 weeks' PRSI contributions paid at Class S in the tax year immediately before the relevant tax year or
- 52 weeks' PRSI contributions paid at Class S in the tax year immediately following the relevant tax year.

If you do not meet these PRSI conditions and you were in insurable employment before becoming self-employed, you may use your PRSI contributions (Class A, E and H) in that employment to qualify for Paternity Benefit – see PRSI conditions for employed people above.

If you are in insurable self-employment, you are not awarded credited contributions or credits automatically when you are getting Paternity Benefit. A self-employed person is not excluded from employment credits specifically. You would however have to satisfy the conditions for credits for employed persons:

- a person must first have entered insurable employment – he or she must have paid at least one PRSI contribution as an employed contributor, and

⏹ a person must, in general, have a paid or credited employment contribution in the previous 2 full tax years. In general where a person has no PRSI paid or credited contributions for two full tax years, they cannot be awarded credits again until they return to work and pay PRSI employment contributions for at least 26 weeks

For example an applicant for Paternity Benefit who is now self-employed but had been employed in 2015 would qualify for credits as they do not have a two-year gap. If they have been only self-employed for the last three years they won't qualify for credits.

Does social insurance outside Ireland count?

If you were previously insurably employed in a country covered by EU Regulations or in a country with which Ireland has a Bilateral Social Security Agreement and you have paid at least one full rate PRSI contribution in Ireland, you may combine your insurance record in that country with your Irish PRSI contributions to help you qualify for Paternity Benefit. You must be in insurable employment in Ireland currently and have paid your most recent PRSI contribution in Ireland.

Can a parent receive Paternity Benefit if the mother and child are resident in another EU member state?

Yes, a parent can receive Paternity Benefit if the mother and child are resident in another EU member state or resident in the European Economic Area (EEA) providing, if employed, they are eligible for Paternity Leave and satisfy the qualifying conditions for Paternity Benefit. If they are self-employed, they will have to self-certify that they are entitled to Paternity Leave and satisfy the qualifying conditions for the Paternity Benefit scheme.

I'm not with the child's mother any more. Can someone else claim the Paternity Benefit?

Only persons defined as a 'relevant parent' are entitled to apply for Paternity Benefit. These are:

- the spouse, civil partner or cohabitant as the case may be of the mother of the child;

- in the case of a child who is being adopted, the spouse, civil partner or cohabitant as the case may be of the adopting mother or sole male adopter; or

- the father of the child

Please note that with the exception of adoption, Paternity Benefit can only be paid once in respect of each child.

Do I have to be living with the mother to be entitled to the benefit?
No.

Can I get another social welfare payment as well as my Paternity Benefit?
You may get half-rate Paternity Benefit if you are getting any of the following payments:

- One-Parent Family Payment

- Widow's, Widower's or Surviving Civil Partner Contributory Pension

- Widow's, Widower's or Surviving Civil Partner Non-Contributory Pension

- Death Benefit by way of Widow's, Widower's, Surviving Civil Partner's or Dependent Parent(s) Pension (under the Occupational Injuries Scheme).

Half-rate Carer's Allowance: If you are providing full-time care to another person, you may also qualify for a half-rate Carer's Allowance along with a standard rate Paternity Benefit. For more information, log on to www.welfare.ie.

Can I get paid my Paternity Benefit if I go to another country?

You will not be paid Paternity Benefit for any period you spend outside the European Economic Area (EEA). If you are an EU citizen, you can get Paternity Benefit for any period of your Paternity Leave spent in an EEA country. If you are not an EU citizen, you will only get Paternity Benefit for any period you spend in the Republic of Ireland.

If you intend to leave the EEA for any period of your paid Paternity Benefit, you must inform Paternity Benefit Section.

Can I be disqualified from receiving Paternity Benefit?

You will be disqualified from receiving Paternity Benefit under the following circumstances:

- If you engage in any form of insurable employment or insurable self-employment during the period for which Paternity Benefit is payable.

- For any period of time spent outside the EEA during the period for which benefit is payable.

- Failure to apply for Paternity Benefit within six months of the birth – or, in the case of adoption, the date of placement – of the child may result in loss of benefit.

What happens if my child is premature?

In the case of a premature birth (before your Paternity Leave is due to start), you should inform the Paternity Benefit section, enclosing your PPS number and written confirmation from a registered medical practioner of the date of birth and the original due date.

What happens if my child is stillborn?

If your child is stillborn after the 24th week of pregnancy, you are entitled to two weeks' Paternity Leave. You may also be entitled to two weeks' paid Paternity Benefit provided you satisfy the social insurance (PRSI) requirements. In addition to a completed Paternity

Benefit application form, you should enclose written confirmation of the original due date, the date your baby was stillborn and the number of weeks' gestation.

My baby did not arrive on the expected due date, how does this affect my Paternity Benefit?
Under legislation Paternity Leave must begin on or after the actual date of birth, or, in the case of adoption, the date of placement and within 26 weeks of that date. If your baby does not arrive on the expected due date please contact your employer in order to select another date on which Paternity Leave can commence. Should you wish to defer your Paternity Benefit payment please contact the Paternity Benefit section on 1890 66 22 44.

My wife wants to spend as long as possible with our new baby. Can I transfer the Paternity Benefit to her?
No.

Can I qualify for Credits while I am getting Paternity Benefit?
If you are in insurable employment and are awarded Paternity Benefit from the Department of Employment Affairs and Social Protection, credits will be automatically added to your record for the period that the benefit is paid to you (up to a maximum of 2 weeks).

If you are in insurable self-employment, you are not awarded credited contributions or credits automatically when you are getting Paternity Benefit. A self-employed person is not excluded from employment credits specifically. You would however have to satisfy the conditions for credits for employed persons –

- a person must first have entered insurable employment – he or she must have paid at least one PRSI contribution as an employed contributor, and

- a person must, in general, have a paid or credited employment contribution in the previous two full tax years.

In general where a person has no PRSI paid or credited contributions for two full tax years, they cannot be awarded credits again until they return to work and pay PRSI employment contributions for at least 26 weeks.

For example an applicant for Paternity Benefit who is now self-employed but had been employed in 2015 would qualify for credits as they does not have a two-year gap. If they have been only self-employed for the last three years they won't qualify for credits.

Am I still entitled to Paternity Leave credits even if I am not entitled to Paternity Benefit?

If you are in insurable employment and not entitled to Paternity Benefit from the Department of Employment Affairs and Social Protection, but you take Paternity Leave from your employment, you will be entitled to have credits added to your record for the period of your Paternity Leave. In this case, you must provide written confirmation from your employer of the periods of Paternity Leave for which you wish to apply for credit, after you return to work.

Can I work while getting Paternity Benefit?

Voluntary work, public representative work (for example Councillor or TD), and courses of education are allowed while you are in receipt of Paternity Benefit. However, you may not engage in insurable (paid) employment or insurable (paid) self-employment and your Paternity Benefit payment will be stopped if you do so.

If you intend to return to work earlier than you had stated on your application form, you must notify the Paternity Benefit Section before your new 'return-to-work date'.

Can I postpone Paternity Benefit?

Paternity Benefit cannot be postponed or delayed except in the case of your child being hospitalised. In all other cases, Paternity Leave must begin on or after the actual date of birth, or, in the case of adoption, the date of placement and within 26 weeks of that date.

For more information on Paternity Benefit contact:

Paternity Benefit Section, Department of Employment Affairs and Social Protection, McCarter's Road, Buncrana, Co. Donegal

Or your local Intreo Centre, Social Welfare Office or Citizen Information Centre.

Or Locall: 1890 66 22 44

www.welfare.ie/paternitybenefit

For information about employment rights and responsibilities, including Paternity Leave, contact:

Workplace Relations Customer Service, Department of Jobs, Enterprise and Innovation, O'Brien Road, Carlow

LoCall: 1890 80 80 90 (from the Republic of Ireland only)

+353 59 917 8990 (from Northern Ireland or overseas)

www.workplacerelations.ie

Parental Leave

The Parental Leave Act 1998, as amended by the Parental Leave (Amendment) Act 2006, allows parents to take parental leave from employment in respect of certain children. A person acting in loco parentis with respect to an eligible child is also eligible.

Duration of parental leave

Since 8 March 2013 the amount of parental leave available for each child amounts to a total of 18 working weeks per child. Where an employee has more than one child, parental leave is limited to 18 weeks in a 12-month period. This can be longer if the employer agrees. Parents of twins or triplets can take more than 18 weeks of parental leave in a year.

The 18 weeks per child may be taken in one continuous period or in two separate blocks of a minimum of six weeks. There must be a gap of at least ten weeks between the two periods of parental leave per child. However, if your employer agrees, you can separate your leave into periods of days or even hours.

Both parents have an equal separate entitlement to parental leave. Unless you and your partner work for the same employer, you can only claim your own parental leave entitlement (18 weeks per child). If you both work for the same employer and your employer agrees, you may transfer fourteen weeks of your parental leave entitlement to each other.

Age of child

Leave can be taken in respect of a child no later than the child's eighth birthday. If a child was adopted between the age of six and eight, leave in respect of that child may be taken up to two years after the date of the adoption order. In the case of a child with a disability or a long-term illness leave may be taken up to 16 years of age.

Illness of parent

If the parent becomes ill while on parental leave the leave can be suspended for the duration of the illness. During the illness the parent is treated as an employee who is sick.

Employment rights while on parental leave

You are not entitled to pay from your employer while you are on parental leave nor are you entitled to any social welfare payment equivalent to Maternity Benefit or Adoptive Benefit. While on parental leave, you must be regarded for employment rights purposes as still working.

Taking parental leave does not affect other employment rights you have. Apart from the loss of pay and pension contributions, your position remains as if no parental leave had been taken. The legislation only provides for the minimum entitlement. Your contract may give you more extensive rights.

Social insurance contributions

The Minister for Social Protection introduced regulations to ensure preservation of social insurance (PRSI) records for employees who take parental leave.

The fine print of parental leave

Generally you must have been working for your employer for a year before you are entitled to parental leave.

If you change job and have used part of your parental leave allowance you can use the remainder after one year's employment with your new employer, provided your child is still under the qualifying age.

Apart from a refusal on the grounds of non-entitlement, an employer may also postpone the leave for up to six months.

Parental leave is to be used only to take care of the child concerned. If the parental leave is taken and used for another purpose the employer is entitled to cancel the leave.

You are entitled to return to your job after your parental leave unless it is not reasonably practicable for the employer to allow you to return to your old job. If this is the case you must be offered a suitable alternative on terms no less favourable compared with the previous job including any improvement in pay or other conditions which occurred while you were on parental leave.

The legislation protects parents who take parental leave from unfair dismissal.

Since 8 March 2013, when you return to work after taking parental leave, you are entitled to ask for a change in your work pattern or working hours for a set period. Your employer must consider your request but is not obliged to grant it.

You must give written notice to your employer of your intention to take parental leave. You should inform your employer in writing at least six weeks before the leave is due to start. The notice should state the starting date and how long the leave will last. After this not less than four weeks before the leave is due to start, you will need to sign a document with your employer confirming the details of the leave.

There are also times when you may require leave or time off work for specific reasons:

Force Majeure Leave

If you have a family crisis the Parental Leave Acts 1998 and 2006 give an employee a limited right to leave from work. This is known as force majeure leave. It arises where, for urgent family reasons, the immediate presence of the employee is indispensable owing to an injury or illness of a close family member. Force majeure leave does not give any entitlement to leave following the death of a close family member.

The maximum amount of leave is three days in any 12-month period or five days in a 36-month period. You are entitled to be paid while you are on force majeure leave. Your employer may grant you further leave.

You are protected against unfair dismissal for taking force majeure leave or proposing to take it. You must notify your employer as soon as practicably possible that you need to avail of force majeure leave. Immediately on your return to work, you must make your application in writing to your employer. Your contract of employment may require you to provide a medical certificate.

As with parental leave, your employer must keep records of all force majeure leave taken by employees.

 For further information log on to:
www.workplacerelations.ie

Maternity Leave

Fathers are entitled to maternity leave if the mother dies within 40 weeks of the birth. In these circumstances, the father is entitled to a period of leave, the extent of which depends on the actual date of the mother's death.

Maternity Benefit is a payment made to women who are on maternity leave from work and covered by social insurance (PRSI). Some employers will continue to pay an employee, in full, while she is on maternity leave and require her to have any Maternity Benefit paid to them. Maternity Benefit is paid for 26 weeks (156 days) at a standard weekly rate. An additional 16 weeks' unpaid maternity leave may be taken, which begins immediately after the end of maternity leave.

iDad: **CLASS ACT**

Under the Maternity Protection (Time off for Antenatal Classes) Regulations 2004, expectant fathers have a once-off right to paid time off work to attend the two antenatal classes immediately prior to the birth.

For further information log on to:
www.citizensinformation.ie
www.welfare.ie

Unmarried Dads and Guardianship Rights

So you are a dad! Not married? That's okay; in this day and age of equality, all things are equal between parents. Aren't they? 'My name is on the baby's birth certificate, so that makes everything equal between us parents. We both have equal rights over the baby. Right?' Wrong.

The following information is provided by Treoir – the National

Specialist Information Service for unmarried parents and their children, which provides clear and up-to-date information free of charge to parents who are not married to each other and to those involved with them.

What is Guardianship?

Guardianship rights allow you to make the major decisions in a child's life – what religion they have, what school they go to, where they live, consenting to their medical treatment, adoption, allowing them to travel.

Am I a guardian?

When a baby is born to an unmarried mother she has full guardianship rights over the baby – automatically. By virtue of giving birth she gets these rights. Many unmarried fathers think because a father's name is on his child's birth certificate that this gives them immediate joint guardianship rights with the mother. It doesn't.

Many fathers think because they may be living with the mother of their child that they have joint guardianship rights*. They don't.

Having your name on your baby's birth certificate says, in a public document, that you are the father of your child. It does not give you any guardianship rights in respect of your child, even if you are living with the mother. This is a common misconception.

How does an unmarried father get guardianship rights?

I. By agreement with the mother

A father and mother can complete and sign the statutory declaration for joint guardianship (S.I. No 5 of 1998). This form declares that:

- the parents have not married each other
- they are the parents of the child, and
- they agree to the appointment of the father as a guardian.

The S.I. No 5 of 1998 form can be downloaded from Treoir's website or ordered from Treoir on 01-6700120 or LoCall 1890 252 084.

When this form is signed and witnessed, it needs to be kept in a safe place as it is the only evidence that the father is a guardian. There is no central register for these Statutory Declarations.

2. By satisfying the cohabitation period*

A father who lives with the child's mother for at least 12 consecutive months including not less than three months after the child's birth, will automatically be the guardian of his child. The three months period does not have to take place directly after the birth of the child. It can be fulfilled any time before the child turns 18 provided that it is part of the 12 consecutive months during which the parents have lived together. The cohabitation period can only be calculated going forward from the commencement date of the Children and Family Relationships Act 2015. This means that guardianship will only be acquired automatically where parents live together for at least 12 months after 18 January 2016.

A declaration that a person is (or is not) a guardian can be applied for through the courts if there is uncertainty, or disagreement, as to whether or not the father has been cohabiting for the required length of time. The application can be made by a guardian of the child or by the person wishing to seek a declaration that they are or are not a guardian of the child. The court shall make a declaration where it is proved on the balance of probabilities that the person named is or is not a guardian of the child.

3. By going to court

The father can apply to the local District Court to become a joint guardian of his child, whether or not his name is on his child's birth certificate. While the mother's views are taken into account by the court in making a decision, the fact that she may not consent does not mean that the court will refuse an order for guardianship. The decision of the court will be made with the best interests of the child being the first and most important consideration. If you are not happy with a decision made by the court you have fourteen days in which to appeal. The terms of the order will come into force while waiting for the appeal unless a court directs otherwise.

4. By getting married following the birth

If the parents of a child marry each other following the birth of their child, then the father automatically becomes a joint guardian.

If a parent (who is a guardian) marries someone other than the parent of the child, his/her spouse will not have an automatic legal relationship to the child. However, the spouse can apply for (limited) guardianship rights if she/he has shared the responsibility of the day-to-care of the child for at least two years.

The only way the spouse can have full legal rights in relation to the child is through adoption. This is called 'step-parent adoption'. If the child is adopted by the parent and his/her spouse, the other biological parent will lose all legal rights in relation to the child.

For further information log on to:
www.treoir.ie or LoCall 1890 252 084

WHAT THE EXPERT SAYS: **WAKE-UP CALL FOR UNMARRIED FATHERS**

The decision of the High Court in the case of JMcB v LE was described at the time (April 2010) as a wake-up call for unmarried fathers of young children. The outcome of this case demonstrated that unless unmarried fathers take the simple step necessary to give legal recognition to their relationship with their children, they could risk being denied contact with their children in circumstances where it is too late to do anything about it.

Unmarried fathers have rights and one very basic and easily protected one, in particular; but in this case the father hadn't exercised it.

The judge in this case found that while the mother's actions could be strongly criticised, the father had not had himself appointed a guardian and therefore the mother had not broken the law.

It is a basic right and, indeed, responsibility of any father who cares about his relationship with his child that he be appointed the child's guardian. Married fathers are automatically guardians of their children.

And it is not simply fathers who should be concerned about ensuring that they are appointed guardians of their children. For a mother in a stable and secure relationship with the father of her children to whom she is not married, she should also be concerned to see that he is appointed a guardian as, if anything were to happen to her, in the absence of a declaration by the mother it may require an application to court to have a legally recognised guardian appointed on behalf of the children.

The appointment of a father as guardian is a simple and straightforward procedure that any unmarried father who takes his relationship with his children seriously should do.

Florence McCarthy LLM, AITI, TEP of McCarthy & Co. Solicitors, Clonakilty, Cork.

iDad: **'MOTHERLESS' PATERNITY TESTING**

Paternity DNA testing seeks to establish whether a man is the true biological father of a child. Performing a paternity test without the mother being involved is possible. Including the mother for testing is always encouraged, but the final decision is left up to the participants to decide.

In many cases the mother is unavailable or chooses not

to participate in the paternity testing process. This does not mean that you cannot still perform the test. A sample from the mother can help increase the accuracy of test results, but conclusive results can still be achieved without her DNA sample.

A person will inherit their DNA from their father and their mother equally. Without the mother's DNA the child's DNA can be compared to the father's DNA. The process and the test performed is no different than when including the mother. This type of paternity test will also be referred to as a motherless paternity testing.

 For further information log on to:
www.easydna.ie

Registering the Birth

Choosing the right name for your baby is extremely important and that is why you are given up to three months to decide to register the name after your baby is born.

Every parent has a legal duty to register the birth of their child. Birth certificates are required for various reasons, eg applying for a passport, school enrolment, health or social welfare applications.

It is also worth noting that when a birth is registered the details are sent directly to the Child Benefit section of the Department of Community Social and Family Affairs and the child benefit is processed automatically. If it is your first child, a partially completed application will be posted to you.

Married parents may register the birth from the maternity hospital, but may still have to visit their local Registrar for Births, Deaths and Marriages to sign the register. They must provide proof of their civilly recognised marriage, by producing a copy of their marriage certificate. Where the marriage occurred outside of the state and the certificate is not in English the parents must provide a certified translation of the full text of the certificate, accompanied by the original.

The registration of stillborn children takes place in the same way as registering a live birth. The staff in your maternity hospital can advise you. If you have adopted a baby, whether from Ireland or overseas, registration will be processed by the Adoption Board.

The **Gender Recognition Act 2015** came into effect on 4 September 2015 and provides that a person can apply for a Gender Recognition Certificate in order to have their preferred gender recognised by the State. The Act also provides for them to apply for a certified copy of an entry in the Register of Gender Recognition. A certificate issued from the Register of Gender Recognition is the equivalent of a birth certificate and satisfies all requirements where a person is asked to provide a birth certificate.

Unmarried parents and birth registration

In Ireland, if the parents of a child are not married to each other, there is no presumption in law as to who is the father of the child, unless the father's name is on the birth certificate. There are different options within Irish registration, relating to the father's details, where the mother and father are not married:

- Both parents can register the birth together by going to the registrar in the hospital or local office (Form CRA 9).

- The mother can complete a declaration form naming the father (Form CRA 1) and bring it along with a declaration by the child's father (Form CRA 3) acknowledging that he is the father of the child. The declaration must be correctly witnessed. The mother then signs the register.

- The father can complete a declaration form acknowledging that he is the father of the child (Form CRA 2) and bring it to the Registrar Office himself. He must also bring with him a declaration by the mother, correctly witnessed, naming him as the father (Form CRA 4).

⌗ The mother or father may make a written request (Form CRA 5 and Form CRA 6 respectively) on production of a certified copy of a court order that names the person to be registered as the father (eg access, maintenance or guardianship). The parent making the request will be required to attend at the Office of the Registrar to sign the Register of Births.

iDad: **LOVE IS ALL AROUND**

In May 2015, Ireland became the first country in the world to bring in same-sex marriage by a popular vote, 62.1% to 37.9%. Just under two million people came out to vote, the highest in any referendum since the foundation of the State – until the vote to repeal the Eighth Amendment in 2018, that is.

Sign of the Times

Following the amendment of the Civil Registration Act of 2014, if a mother attends without the father to register her child's birth the Registrar will register the birth without a surname for the child and without the father's details. The mother will be asked for contact details of the father and the Registrar will then make 'all reasonable efforts' to contact the father and invite him to attend the Registrar's Office within 28 days in order to complete the registration. Only in exceptional cases, where 'compelling reasons' are provided, will the father's name be omitted.

Re-Registration

If the child has been registered in the mother's name alone, it is possible to re-register the birth at any future date in order to have the father's details included, using any of the methods outlined above for registration.

For additional information log on to:
www.treoir.ie
www.citizensinformation.ie
www.ihrec.ie
www.welfare.ie

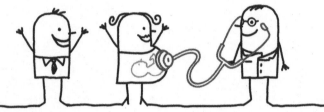

'A grand adventure is about
to begin.'

Winnie the Pooh

8 What's up, Doc?

The glossary

In the unlikely event that you are brave enough to ask a question during the antenatal visit, or if you plan on sitting in on the baby shower with all the other blooming belles, then it is best advised that you become familiar with a few of the words, terms and phrases that will most likely pop up during the pregnancy ...

Afterbirth: The afterbirth is another name for the placenta and foetal membranes which are delivered 'after the birth' of your baby.

Alpha fetoprotein (AFP): Alpha-fetoprotein (AFP) is a protein found in all foetuses. The AFP test is a blood test used to check the baby for any abnormalities or birth defects.

Amniocentesis: Amniocentesis is a test in which a small amount of fluid is collected from the pregnancy sac around the baby in the womb to look for any birth defects and chromosome problems including Down Syndrome.

Amniotic fluid: The amniotic fluid surrounds and protects the baby during pregnancy.

Amniotic sac: The bag which holds the fluid located inside the uterus, where the baby develops and grows.

Anaemia: Anaemia is caused by low levels of red blood cells. Iron deficiency is the most common form which can affect the growth of the baby.

Anti-D (see **Rhesus Factor**)**:** Anti-D is given to prevent pregnant women who have a rhesus negative blood group from producing antibodies against their rhesus positive foetus.

Apgar test: An Apgar test is given following the birth. The baby's appearance, heartbeat, reflex response, muscle tone and breathing are checked.

Baby Blues: After the birth of a baby, approximately half of all new mums suffer a period of mild depression called the 'blues'. This may last for a few hours or, at most, for a few days before disappearing.

BCG (Bacille Calmette-Guérin): The BCG vaccination is usually given to newborn babies, but can also be given to older children and adults who are considered to be at risk of developing Tuberculosis.

Birth canal: The birth canal is the passage between the vaginal opening and cervix, or in other words, the vagina.

Birth plan: A written record of what your partner would like to happen during labour and after the baby is born.

Braxton Hicks: Braxton Hicks contractions help your partner's uterus 'practise' for upcoming labour.

Breech birth: A breech birth is when the baby is born either feet or bottom first, instead of the normal head first.

Caesarean section/C-section: A C-section is a surgical procedure to deliver the baby through an incision in your partner's lower abdomen. C-sections are often conducted when unexpected problems arise during the delivery.

Carpal tunnel syndrome: Carpal tunnel syndrome (CTS) is a relatively common condition that occurs in pregnancy which causes pain, numbness and a burning or tingling sensation in the hand and fingers.

Cervix: The cervix is the lower portion of the uterus which widens (dilates) during childbirth to allow the baby to pass through.

Chorionic villus sampling (CVS): CVS is a test conducted to identify chromosome abnormalities and other inherited disorders involving the removal of some chorionic villi cells from the placenta, where it attaches itself to the uterine wall.

Clots: After giving birth, it is normal for your partner to experience bleeding for a short period. Often, this bleeding will be accompanied by blood clots. Blood clots that appear after childbirth are part of a healing process known as lochia (postpartum bleeding).

Colostrum: A form of milk loaded with nutrients and antibodies produced in late pregnancy and the few days following childbirth which keeps newborn babies strong and healthy.

Contraction: A contraction is the tightening of the upper uterine muscle that 'contracts' the size of the uterus, pushing the baby towards the birth canal.

Cot death: Cot death, also referred to as sudden infant death syndrome (SIDS), is the sudden unexpected death of an infant.

Couvade syndrome: Couvade syndrome, or sympathetic pregnancy, is when an expectant father experiences some of the physical symptoms of pregnancy prior to the baby's birth.

Crowning: Crowning occurs when the baby's head is visible through the vaginal opening.

Dilation: The moment your partner's cervix begins to open and thin out prior to your baby being born.

Doppler: A Doppler is a device that allows you to listen to the baby's heartbeat.

Doula: A doula, or birth attendant, refers to someone who offers emotional and physical support to a pregnant woman and her partner before, during and after childbirth.

Down syndrome: A condition caused by chromosomal abnormalities which leads to impairments in both learning ability and physical growth. It can be detected through a series of screenings and tests before the baby is born (see **Amniocentesis & Nuchal Translucency Screening**).

Eclampsia: A pregnant woman who has been previously diagnosed with **pre-eclampsia** (see below) develops seizures or coma.

Ectopic pregnancy: An ectopic pregnancy is a pregnancy that occurs outside a pregnant woman's uterus.

EDD: Expected Date of Delivery.

Effacement: Effacement pertains to the thinning and softening of the cervix.

Embryo: An embryo refers to an unborn baby in the first eight weeks following implantation.

Entonox: Entonox is a mix of nitrous oxide 50 per cent and oxygen 50 per cent, or **Gas & Air**, often used as a method of pain relief in labour.

Engagement: Engagement is a term used to describe when the baby enters the pelvis in preparation for the delivery.

Engorgement: Breast engorgement is the overfilling of the breasts with milk.

Epidural: A common method of pain relief in labour, an epidural analgesia refers to the process in which anaesthesia is injected into a part of the spine known as the epidural space.

Episiotomy: A surgical cut that is sometimes necessary to enlarge the vaginal opening to help deliver the baby.

External cephalic version (ECV): The movement of a breech baby into the head-first position.

Fallopian tube: The fallopian tubes are a pair of thin tubes connecting the ovaries to the uterus. In reproduction an egg is released from the ovary and travels along the fallopian tube and into the uterus.

Foetus: A foetus describes a baby after eight weeks of development.

Fontanelle: Commonly referred to as a soft spot on a baby's head, the fontanelle allows the baby's head pass easily through the birth canal.

Forceps: A surgical tool used to assist in the delivery of the baby which resembles a large pair of pincers or tweezers.

Gas & Air: See 'Entonox'.

Gestation: Gestation is the period of development of a baby inside the womb.

Heel-prick test: The heel prick or Guthrie test is conducted between six days and two weeks after birth, by which time the baby will be well established on milk feeds. Blood is collected by pricking the baby's heel which is analysed for conditions such as cystic fibrosis, hypothyroidism and phenylketonuria (PKU).

Human chorionic gonadotropin (hCG): hCG is a hormone that is produced by the placenta of a pregnant woman which is detectable in the blood and urine within ten days of fertilisation.

Induction: Induction of labour denotes commencing the labour contractions with medical procedures, as opposed to waiting for labour to occur naturally.

In vitro fertilisation (IVF): IVF is the process of fertilising eggs with sperm outside of the human body.

Jaundice: 'Newborn jaundice' is a condition marked by high levels of bilirubin in the blood. The increased bilirubin causes the infant's skin and whites of the eyes to appear yellowish. Usually disappears between 7–10 days following the birth.

Labour: The process by which the birth occurs, beginning with contractions of the uterus and ending with the delivery of the baby, followed by the placenta.

Lactation: Lactation refers to the secretion or production of breast milk.

Lanugo: The lanugo is the fine, soft hair covering the body of a foetus and newborn.

Latch: Latch is a term to describe how a baby attaches itself to the breast while feeding.

Male postnatal depression: Although postnatal depression in a man is not hormonal, it is said to be brought on by the new pressures of fatherhood. It can also occur if the mother is going through her own battle with postnatal depression.

Mastitis: Mastitis is an infection that commonly affects women who are breastfeeding.

Meconium: Meconium, or baby pooh, is a thick, green, tar-like substance that lines your baby's intestines during pregnancy and is released in your baby's first bowel movements after the birth.

Midwife: A midwife is a health professional who provides pregnancy, birth and postnatal support for expectant mums.

Miscarriage: Miscarriage is defined as the loss of pregnancy before the 20th week.

Morning sickness: Morning sickness is the nausea and vomiting associated with pregnant women. It is caused by the sudden increase in hormones, and though more common in the morning, it can strike at any time of the day.

Nappy rash: Nappy rash is a very common condition which can occur when a baby's skin is exposed to a wet, or dirty, nappy for too long, resulting in the baby's skin becoming sore, red, and tender.

Nesting: Nesting refers to the powerful urge to prepare the home for the baby.

Nuchal translucency screening: An ultrasound is taken to measure the translucent area in the skin on the back of the baby's neck (the nuchal fold), to determine whether there is a risk of the baby developing a chromosomal abnormality, such as Down syndrome.

Obstetrician: An obstetrician is a medical specialist who takes care of pregnant women from the time of conception, through to childbirth and the immediate postnatal period afterwards.

Oestrogen: Oestrogen is a hormone which is secreted by the ovaries.

Ovulation: Ovulation occurs when a mature egg is released from the ovary, pushed down the fallopian tube, and made available for fertilisation.

Oxytocin: Oxytocin is a hormone which causes the contraction of the uterus during labour and stimulates the ejection of milk into the ducts of the breasts.

Perineum: The perineum is the area from the anus to the vaginal opening, where an episiotomy is performed.

Pethidine: Pethidine, comparable to morphine and a member of the family of drugs known as opioids, is a drug widely used for pain relief in labour.

Placenta: The placenta, or afterbirth, is an organ that forms inside of the womb during pregnancy which helps to nourish the baby.

Placenta praevia: Placenta praevia occurs when the placenta implants itself very low in the womb covering all or part of the internal opening of the cervix.

Polycystic ovary syndrome: PCOS is a hormonal imbalance found in women which can cause infertility. Polycystic ovaries are unable to produce the normal levels of hormones required to release one egg at ovulation each month.

Postnatal depression/postpartum depression (PPD): Unlike the 'baby blues', postnatal depression is a long-term clinical condition which affects women after childbirth.

Pre-eclampsia: Pre-eclampsia is a condition in pregnancy which results in high blood pressure, water retention and protein in your urine (see **eclampsia**).

Quickening: Quickening refers to the first time the baby is felt moving.

Rhesus factor: Everybody's blood is either rhesus positive or rhesus negative. When an expectant mum is Rh negative and her baby is Rh positive, there may be health implications for the baby (see **Anti-D**).

Show: The release of a blood-tinged mucous plug from the cervix when labour is imminent.

SIDS: Sudden Infant Death Syndrome (see **Cot death**).

Stillbirth: A stillbirth is the death of a baby after the 20th week of pregnancy but before delivery.

Stretch marks: Marks in the skin that appear in the later stages of pregnancy when the belly is expanding to accommodate the growing baby.

Transcutaneous electrical nerve stimulation: A TENS Machine is a common method of pain relief in labour. A special device transmits low-voltage electrical impulses through electrodes on the skin to the area of the body that is in pain.

Toxoplasmosis: Toxoplasmosis is an infection that comes from parasites found in cats' faeces and undercooked meat which can prove to be fatal to an unborn baby.

Transition: Transition is the stage of labour prior to when the delivery begins. During this phase, the cervix will dilate from 7 to 10cm.

Trimester: The word trimester means 'three months'.

Ultrasound: An ultrasound uses high-frequency sound waves to produce images of a baby.

Umbilical cord: The umbilical cord connects the baby in the womb to its mother. It transports nutrients to the baby and also carries away the baby's waste products. It is made up of three blood vessels: two arteries and one vein.

Uterus: A female organ located in the pelvis above the vagina, more commonly known as the **womb**.

Ventouse extraction: A ventouse (vacuum extractor) is an instrument that uses suction to attach a soft rubber or metal cup on to the baby's head which is attached to a suction device. Once the baby's head is born, the cup is removed and the baby's body is born naturally.

Vernix caseosa: Vernix is a white cheesy substance that covers and protects the skin of the baby in the womb.

Womb: See **Uterus**.

Zygote: A zygote is the medical term given to a fertilised egg.

Leabharlanna Poiblí Chathair Baile Átha Cliath
Dublin City Public Libraries

Useful Resources
Irish Parenting & Forum Websites

For him ... **Dad.ie**

For her ...

www.eumom.ie

www.magicmum.com

www.mummypages.ie

www.mams.ie

www.rollercoaster.ie

General

A Little Lifetime Foundation (formerly Isands) **www.alittlelifetime.ie**

Association for Improvements in the Maternity Services **www.aimsireland.ie**

Aware – Helping to beat Depression **www.aware.ie**

Citizens Information Board **www.citizensinformation.ie**

Cuidiu – Irish Childbirth Trust **www.cuidiu-ict.ie**

Doula Ireland **www.doulaireland.com**

Down Syndrome Ireland **www.downsyndrome.ie**

Equality Authority **www.ihrec.ie**

Equal shared parenting rights & responsibilities: **www.irishdads.ie**

Friends of Breastfeeding **www.friendsofbreastfeeding.ie**

Homebirth Association of Ireland **www.homebirth.ie**

Irish Multiple Births Association **www.imba.ie**

Irish Sudden Infant Death Association **www.firstlight.ie**

La Leche League of Ireland **www.lalecheleagueireland.com**

Men's Health Forum in Ireland **www.mhfi.org**

Miscarriage Association of Ireland **www.miscarriage.ie**

Money Advice & Budgeting Service (MABS) **www.mabs.ie**

National Infertility Support & Information Group **www.nisig.ie**

One Family – For One Parent Families **www.onefamily.ie**

Parentline – A Helpline for Parents & Guardians **www.parentline.ie**

Postnatal Depression Ireland **www.pnd.ie**

Solo – Lone Parenting **www.solo.ie**

The National Sudden Infant Death Register **www.sidsireland.ie**

Treoir – Information for Unmarried Parents **www.treoir.ie**

Unmarried & Separated Parents of Ireland **www.uspi.ie**

Suggested Irish Pregnancy titles for Mum-to-be

The Irish Pregnancy Book, Dr Peter Boylan, The O'Brien Press, 2015.

The Better Birth Book, Tracy Donegan, The Liffey Press, 2006.

Hot Cross Mum, Hazel Gaynor, e-book, 2011.

Misadventures in Motherhood, Fiona Looney, O'Brien Press, 2005.

Mum's Guide to Having Your Baby in Ireland, Lucy Taylor, Gill & Macmillan, 2010.

For Couples

Recovering from Postnatal Depression, Madge Fogarty, 2011.

TTC: Trying to Conceive: The Irish Couples Guide, Fiona McPhillips, Liberties Press, 2005.

We Lost our Baby, Siobhan O'Neill-White & David White, The Liffey Press, 2007

References

Passive smoking increases risk to unborn babies
www.nottingham.ac.uk/news/pressreleases/2011/march/
passivesmoking.aspx

Fathers-to-be in Ireland need to lose weight
www.coombe.ie/index.php?nodeId=12&documentId=668&PHPSESSI
D=4b843c7ee7c5504058748dd28ba5269c

More than one in five pregnancies ends in miscarriage
miscarriage.ie/aboutmiscarriage.html

Statistics on Home Births in Ireland
www.homebirth.ie/index.asp?mm=3&msm=1

Central Statistics Office – Irish Baby Names 2017/8
www.cso.ie/en/interactivezone/visualisationtools/babynamesofireland/

www.cso.ie/en/csolatestnews/pressreleases/2017pressreleases/
pressstatementbabynamesofireland/

Ryanair – Expectant Mother – Fitness to Fly
www.ryanair.com/doc/conditions/FR-FITTOFLYLETTERS.pdf

Know the New Law on Child Car Seats
www.rsa.ie/Documents/Road%20Safety/Safety%20for%20kids/
Child%20Safety%20in%20Cars%20English.pdf

If mum is happy and you know it, wave your fetal arms
www.newscientist.com/article/mg20527514.000-if-mum-is-happy-
and-you-know-it-wave-your-fetal-arms.html

Do dummies help prevent SIDS?
www.nct.org.uk/sites/default/files/related_documents/dodds-do-
dummies-help-prevent-sids-20-1-.pdf

WHO 10 Facts on Breastfeeding
www.who.int/features/factfiles/breastfeeding/facts/en/index.html

Safe Food
www.safefood.eu/Publications/Consumer-information/How-to-prepare-your-baby-s-bottle.aspx

What is the Period of Purple Crying?
www.purplecrying.info/sections/index.php?sct=1&

Prenatal and Postpartum Depression in Fathers
jama.ama-assn.org/content/303/19/1961.short

Incidence of Maternal and Paternal Depression in Primary Care
archpedi.ama-assn.org/cgi/content/abstract/2010.184v1

Paternity leave & benefit
www.citizensinformation.ie/en/social_welfare/social_welfare_payments/social_welfare_payments_to_families_and_children/paternity_benefit.html

www.citizensinformation.ie/en/social_welfare/social_welfare_payments/social_welfare_payments_to_families_and_children/paternity_benefit.html

www.welfare.ie/en/Pages/Paternity-Benefit.aspx

Parental leave
www.citizensinformation.ie/en/employment/employment_rights_and_conditions/leave_and_holidays/parental_leave.html

Other types of leave
www.citizensinformation.ie/en/employment/employment_rights_and_conditions/leave_and_holidays/types_of_leave_from_work.html

ESB's 'Life Work Balance' – Paternity leave
www.esbelectricmail.com/_archives/em_archive/archives/november2006_em/news/nov_news22.htm

Equality Authority seeks reform of Family Law to recognise the reality of modern family life
www.equality.ie/index.asp?docID=850

Treoir: Guardianship of Children
http://www.treoir.ie/wp-content/uploads/2018/03/Guardianship-of-children.pdf

Treoir: Registration of Births of Children whose parents are not married to each other
www.treoir.ie/information-registration.php

Contraception choices – Effectiveness of Pill
thinkcontraception.ie/Contraception-Choices/The-Pill-and-Mini-Pill.103.1.aspx

Index